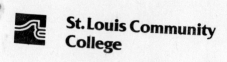

St. Louis Community
College

Library

5801 Wilson Avenue
St. Louis, Missouri 63110

BRO
LAR     PRINTED IN U.S.A.

23-263-002

# Doctor
## and
# child

Books by T. Berry Brazelton, M.D.

INFANTS AND MOTHERS
TODDLERS AND PARENTS
DOCTOR AND CHILD

# Doctor
## and
# child

T. Berry Brazelton, M.D.

*With photographs by Steven Trefonides*

*A Merloyd Lawrence Book*

DELACORTE PRESS / SEYMOUR LAWRENCE

The photograph in Chapter 4, "Colic," is by
Edward Tronick and Denise Zwahlen
Much of the material in this book first appeared in *Redbook*.

Manufactured in the United States of America
Designed by Jerry Tillett
First printing

*Library of Congress Cataloging in Publication Data*

Brazelton, T    Berry, 1918–
Doctor and child.
"A Merloyd Lawrence book."
1. Children—Care and hygiene. 2. Children—
Management. 3. Pediatricians. I. Title.
RJ61.B816 1976     649.1     76–7898

ISBN 0–440–02074–3

To Kitty, Polly, Stina, and Tom

# Acknowledgments

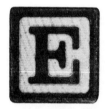ach chapter in this book is
composed of two sections. The first
section of each chapter appeared
as an article in *Redbook* magazine
during the years 1970–74. They
have graciously given them up for
reprinting. The second section of each chapter
was written especially for this book, to bring the
subject up-to-date and emphasize the basic issues
involved. I hope that this expanded format will
make the discussion more useful. I am
particularly indebted to Sey Chassler, editor in
chief of *Redbook* magazine, to Robert Levin, his
associate editor, to Carlo Vittorini, its gifted
publisher, and to Mrs. Katherine Ball Ross for
teaching me to write so that the pedantry of
medical school teaching does not submerge the
reader. My publishers, Seymour and Merloyd
Lawrence, have been offering constant, necessary
encouragement, and Merloyd Lawrence has

brought it to editorial fulfillment. To them I am extremely grateful.

And, last but not least, to my own long-suffering mother, to my wife and children, I offer my belated thanks for allowing me the time and support to attempt this task. My patients in Cambridge over the past twenty-five years have contributed their own expertise to the ideas in this book, and I hope they recognize and bask in whatever success it may have.

# Contents

# Introduction

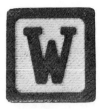hen a young pediatrician finishes hospital training today, he or she is faced with an important decision: whether to pursue an ivory tower kind of career—as a teacher and researcher who sees patients who are referred by other physicians—or whether to take on the demanding role of being the "family doctor" for many patients in private practice. The practice of pediatrics is changing today, away from the overworked, tired, but dedicated physician who made house calls at the end of his twelve-hour day, to a more reasonable type of group practice in which nurse practitioners are often at the forefront of caring for patients, screening them for the physician in order not to "waste his time." I suspect that this changing role will take even more of the reward out of pediatrics for those young men and women whose reason for having become physicians was

the desire to work in a close, meaningful relationship with parents and their children.

What will this do to the practice of pediatrics in the future? Will pediatricians become consultants, seeing young patients only when they are in real trouble? I hope not, for there is nothing more rewarding than the day-to-day relationship which one builds up with young parents as they face the inevitable problems of adjusting to a new infant. Each day, when I return from my teaching and research at the Harvard Medical School, I look forward, as a small child does to his "lovey," or favorite toy, to handling and holding a vital, healthy baby or toddler and to discussing the issues that are met in this book with vital, eager young parents. There is hope, strength, and excitement in a developing child, and the reward for a physician is the chance to play an intimate role in furthering this development.

I have wanted to be a doctor for as long as I can remember. When I used to read of Dr. Doolittle's adventures, I nodded and felt identified with him as he tended his talking animals. The rewards he felt when one of them recovered came back to me when, as an adolescent, I mended the legs of chickens who fell off roosts, stuffed medicine down dogs' throats, and did my best to learn something about veterinary medicine. It turned out to be more complex than I'd expected, and I became impatient to get on to medical school.

Meanwhile, as the oldest grandchild of fourteen in a rather close extended family in Texas, I was given the baby-sitting job for all the younger ones while the adults celebrated Thanksgiving,

Christmas, and other holidays. I found it even more rewarding to comfort an unhappy child than to mend a chicken who was even more afraid of you afterward. I got the same thrill when a small cousin looked up in my face as I rocked her in the big swing chair on Grandma Brazelton's front porch that I do today when I cuddle a new baby to quiet her from crying.

College and medical school seemed to take so long. Much of the curriculum was stuffed with "unimportant" drudgery, such as history, economics, and histology. Even anatomy and pathology seemed so depersonalized that they were hard to study, but they seemed related somewhere to the ultimate goal—of getting on to being a real people's "doctor."

Medical school was a brainwashing experience. All of it seemed depersonalized and disappointing. We finally saw and laid hands on real patients in the third year. But they too were separated from us—by the hospital hierarchy which was really in charge of them, by our inexperience and our anxiety, by the professor who came in to check our work and spoke in front of them as if they were not there. I began to wonder whether this was what I had waited so long for. Patients were looked upon as if their sole purpose in the hospital was to be the host for a disease with which we were concerned—a far cry from Dr. Doolittle's relationships with his patients.

But one began to be numb after a while. The overwhelming number of disease entities, the long lists of symptoms that make up each disease seemed to become the sheep one counts at night as well as the gold one searched for in diagnosing each patient. Feelings of medical students are blunted, and with this blunting, their concern for the feelings of their patients begins to lose priority. Then, when internship with its increased physical demands rolled around, it was a jolt to be brought to realize that one was indeed dealing with people, not diseases.

I remember one eight-year-old boy named Ernie who had chronic kidney disease. Ernie was not only the size of a four-year-old, having been dwarfed by his disease, but he was swollen and puffy and looked like a large, miserable baby. His mother stayed near him a great deal in the hospital, and we rather resented her for it, for she seemed to be a constant reminder that Ernie was not improving. We did not have the answer to a cure for him and we were in the medical racket to cure people. It became harder and harder for us (interns and nurses) to go into Ernie's room at all. Days would pass before we were jogged to go in to see him.

One day, Mrs. Imbruglio, Ernie's mother, asked me what day I would be off duty. She then asked me whether she could have me over to her apartment to eat an Italian dinner with Ernie's family. I was so surprised by the invitation that I said yes, and spent the rest of the day wondering why I'd let myself in for such a thing. As it began to approach the time for dinner, I felt a combination of feelings, dominated by my guilty feelings for not having paid more attention to Ernie. I asked for and received permission to take Ernie along to dinner as a surprise for his family.

Ernie was a soft, cuddly little mass as I carried him up the stairs. He had always whimpered when we handled him in the hospital and we'd left him alone, fearing he was in pain. Now he smiled fetchingly and reached up to tickle my face. When we finally reached the fourth floor and his family's apartment, we were talking to each other and were real friends. Of course, I don't need to describe the Latin emotions that greeted us, as Ernie reveled in their surprise at his visit. I ate so much Italian spaghetti that my stomach ached for days, but Ernie and I remained friends. He smiled understandingly at me when I had to come in to draw blood from him, began to cry only after the needle was inserted, and allowed himself to be comforted by me after it was over. He and I had a different kind of understanding of each other now. When I could break away, I sat with Mrs. Imbruglio. We talked of her family and how much they helped her face Ernie's inevitable outcome, so she could stand to come in day after day to help Ernie with his side of dying. I began to see an entirely new side of medicine, and a new role a physician might play—even when his medicine was no longer able to save the life he wanted so desperately to save. Ernie went gradually downhill and finally into a merciful coma. By teaching me how to become a support for him, his mother and his family were indeed the most important learning experience I had as an intern. The Imbruglios set my course on track again.

I found that even as a busy intern there was time left over to talk to children and their parents

—about themselves and their feelings toward the illness and hospitalization. It took me twenty-two years to get the self-assurance needed to write the article on hospitalization in this book, but my conviction remains firm that children, their families, *and* hospital personnel as well could learn from each other to make an illness and even a hospitalization into a positive rather than negative experience.

After seven years of training to become a qualified pediatrician, I was ready to step out into the world of private practice. But it was too big a step. I knew by then that I was in no way fitted to understand children or their parents, and I was not content to stick to their physical symptoms. At the time that I finished training, there was no way for a physician to learn about people and about problems in development except by taking off for a year or two to train as a psychiatrist. As I told my professor of pediatrics about my decision to do this, he responded with "What a waste of all that good pediatric training!"

Now, over twenty years later, I realize more than ever that medical school training in physiological problems helps a pediatrician only a small part of the time. In a sixty- to seventy-hour week, only 15 percent of my time is spent in doing physical examinations and giving advice about physical symptoms. This 15 percent is fascinating and vital, but it is facilitated by antibiotics, good clinical facilities, and referrals to experts in the appropriate field. The other 85 percent of my time is made up of advice, guidance, and counseling about psychological or developmental problems, what I consider "the art of medicine." A case of "colic" in an infant is far more challenging to a pediatrician these days than a hearty strep throat, and more exciting to treat if it *is* approached as a psychosomatic problem.

Before beginning practice, however, I could only guess at this need for psychological understanding. Fortunately, during my internship, I had a very searching experience: observing the child psychiatrist Dr. Marian Putnam with a three-year-old disturbed child. We at the Massachusetts General Hospital had been unable to make a diagnosis with this mute, Ophelia-like toddler. She literally tore up her bed, destroyed her clothing, pulled out her hair, and we'd resorted to tying her to her bed. None of us could handle her. Dr. Putnam was called in to consult with us. She gathered the child up in her arms, settled into a rocking chair to rock gently, crooning softly to our Ophelia. The child was quiet for the first time in ten days, and even looked pretty and content. All of a sudden, she urinated on Dr. Putnam's lap. I felt responsible and horrified, tried to snatch her away. Dr. Putnam kept on rocking, looked down at the baby, and said, "That's nice. You finally are willing to communicate with me." This kind of understanding acceptance of a disturbed child's behavior was a revelation. I wanted to understand children the way she did.

In the next four years, at a psychiatric unit called the Putnam Children's Center in Boston, I learned how to play with small children—by being a nursery school teacher; how to interview parents—by being a social worker; and, finally, what it meant for young parents and small children to have a therapeutic relationship with a physician—by being a child psychiatrist.

In this period, we started a longitudinal study of normal parents and children to try to understand the mechanisms by which new parents cope with their anxiety about being responsible for new infants. As we studied couples during the woman's pregnancy, we were amazed that they could learn to cope at all. However, I gradually realized that their concerns about whether they could change from adolescents to new parents, their anxious fears about whether their baby might be damaged, became the cornerstone for the intense attachment which they mustered around the new infant after birth. It was my first realization that anxiety could be a very healthy mechanism, mobilizing energy to cope with a new and frightening experience—that of parenting a dependent human being.

But I also began to feel with these young parents the burden of self-questioning that our society places upon them. Somewhere there is a myth that everything that goes wrong with a child is the fault of the parents. The myth goes this way —the infant is born with a potential for perfection. But he or she is like a lump of clay, at the mercy of the environment. And every flaw in the child's upbringing unfits him or her for the competitive society that we all live in. So parents become tense about decision-making before they begin. Children feel their parents' indecision, become anxious themselves, and we are

perpetuating unnecessarily tense generations,
with no joy in each other.

My concern as a pediatrician has been to find
ways to dispel some of this destructive
self-recrimination, to shore up parents so they can
feel more adequate, can even learn to enjoy being
parents. I have been sure that if we could do that,
children would be surer of themselves and of
their families—and we might prevent some of the
developmental problems that beleaguer young
families today.

As I observed new babies in the newborn
nurseries, I realized that they were *not* lumps of
clay, ready to be shaped by the environment. Each
infant was a strong individual at birth. And they
expressed themselves in ways that made it very
clear to parents *who could listen* that they would
best be handled in certain ways, and not in others.
The patterns for childrearing set up by our
society, and by which parents shape their
children might suit a particular child—but they
also might well not. And if parents could be
helped to listen to their infants and respect them
as individuals with strong reactions, they could
have a much better and easier time together. On
the strength of this thesis, I wrote *Infants and
Mothers: Individual Differences in Development.* I
hope it has supported new parents to look for
individuality in their babies, and to enjoy them
from the beginning as vital young personalities.

In the present book, I hope to raise and answer
in more detail many of the common, burning
questions that arise in my practice. I have a
telephone hour at the beginning of each day and a

consultation hour at the end of my office hours. In these two periods, parents ask questions and we discuss the dynamics of the problem—for them and for the child.

These consultations are a form of teamwork; they would be of little value unless parents took the time to put their most important concerns into words. Some parents who read this book may have found their own pediatricians are overloaded with work and not responsive to developmental or psychological problems. This is an area in which parents can influence the medical system. Just as the Childbirth Education Association has pressured obstetricians toward less medication and the father's participation toward a more "natural" kind of childbirth, and influenced hospitals to allow "rooming in," so too can concerned parents press for involvement of pediatricians and family practitioners in the total development of the child. Public demand is a powerful instrument. In the long run this may mean a change in the training of medical personnel.

The suggestions and insights in this book may not offer sufficient answers for any set of parents. But I hope they will furnish the base for thinking about each issue and for further questions from parents to their physicians. The first chapter, "How to Get Along with Your Child's Doctor," is especially intended to encourage parents who lack the courage to turn to their pediatrician.

# Doctor
## and
# child

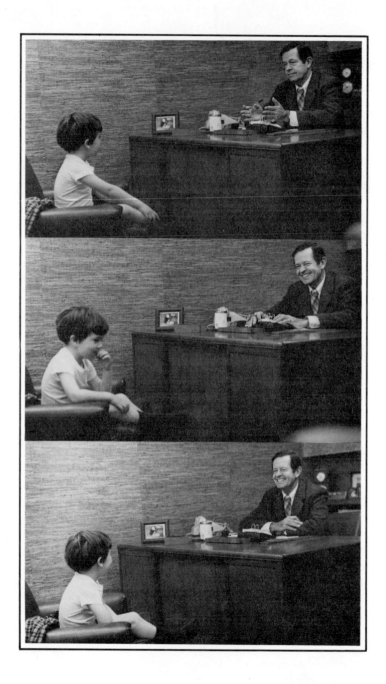

## Chapter 1

# How to get along with your child's doctor

he young mother of today who is competent and efficient takes pride in the way she handles her household. Minor domestic crises leave her unruffled. Still, there are times when she is not so sure of herself. Usually it's a problem that has to do with her child.

She is probably sensitive and aware enough to know that a child's first few years have a profound influence on his or her emotional adjustment later in life. So when her two-year-old shows signs of negativism she is concerned—and she questions her own ability to deal with it. Looking around for guidance, too often she finds there is no place to turn.

Frequently she is not in touch with her family. Her own mother may be either too far away in distance or too far away in thinking. And seldom is the reliability of an extended family—a network of grandparents, aunts, uncles, cousins—available to her. An older, wiser family friend whom she has always counted on for advice may not be there to help her. Instead she finds the harried next-door neighbor who is having problems with her own difficult toddler. True, our young mother finds a certain comfort in comparing notes with her friend on mutual problems, but too soon and too often their exchange ends up in a competition to prove the superiority of their respective children.

Her husband certainly helps her to sort out her thinking about the child, but she has need of another, objective, more authoritative source to rely on. When she is desperate she turns to childrearing literature and how-to-do-it programs on radio and television. But how much more satisfying it would be if she could turn to a *person* who knows about children, someone who could give her and her child individual attention and guidance—how much more satisfying if she could turn to a physician!

Mothers reading this will immediately say, "But where do I find a physician who wants me and my child? The pediatricians in my town are disease-oriented specialists, and they couldn't care less about me and my problems with my children." Or, "They are overworked and have no time."

Having been an overworked, too-busy pediatrician for twenty years, I know what you are saying and how true it is. Perhaps I am being idealistic, as I write this, in talking about a rare, difficult-to-find entity—a satisfying relationship among parents, their child, and the pediatrician. And the tragic thing to me is that it will be even rarer and more difficult to find in the next ten years.

Quite probably we will see the solo practice of pediatrics vanish, to be replaced by groups of doctors in clinics, where parents must relate to whomever they happen to reach. Nurse practitioners will become the confidants and advisers of the young parents, and the pediatrician will be reserved only for serious physical illness. This will make it even more difficult for the mother and father, the physician and child, to find their way in setting up the kind of relationship I want to talk about. Still, I think such a relationship is possible even with all the difficulties that do exist.

Especially is it possible if you bear in mind one thing: The relationship between parents and pediatrician has one major goal—the well-being of the child. At the same time it is a working partnership that carries important responsibilities for each of the participants. When mother, father, and pediatrician take their own side of the relationship seriously and communicate well with one another, a fruitful and rewarding relationship will surely follow.

Let me explain what I mean with an example from my own practice. I remember a mother who called me daily for several weeks with questions about her infant, and when I tired of her overdependency, as I thought it, and suggested that she figure out some of these things for herself, she stopped phoning during the regular morning call hour. But she punished me by having her husband ring me in the middle of the night with all her stored-up questions, thinly couched in a plea for help with the baby's loose bowel movements, not at all a serious condition.

Then I realized that this poor mother was not getting from me the kind of help she needed and she was angry about it. My inclination had been to "fire" her as a patient. Instead we discussed how unsatisfactory—for each of us—our relationship had become. As we talked she disclosed some of the insecure feelings she had as a mother, and I understood that her demanding attitude was her way of asking for my help.

Our talk gave me new tools as her doctor. I gained, first of all, a better understanding of her as a person, then an insight into the ways I could work with her as a mother, and finally a warmer, more protective feeling for her as "my" patient.

Further, I was able to make positive suggestions about improving our relationship. I informed her that there were other sources—her husband, her own mother, her friends, perhaps even a community-service nurse—to whom she could turn for support, and indicated how these people might be of help to her. Of course, I stressed that I was certainly available when she really needed me, and said that if she would call during the morning call hour, she would find me with energy enough to help her. Also I asked that when she did need my help, she express her need and her problem directly so that I would not have the feeling of being "had."

With this new, better-understood relationship,

we have worked well together, and her three children are among my most cherished patients. She claims that she grew up with our discussions. I did too.

Of course, the one who will profit most from the parents' relationship with the doctor is the child. Not only will he or she have better physical care because parents and pediatrician communicate well, but also he or she will sense the basic trust that exists in a good working relationship.

Young parents who have been afraid of their own doctors as they grew up may find it hard not to transfer old fears and anxiety to their children. By the same token, a mother or father who *expects* to have a good relationship with a physician transmits this trust to the child. In times of crisis—such as those surrounding illnesses or inoculations—when any child hates being looked at or poked at, such parents can reassure their child. By doing this they certainly make my job easier—and they also help their child by easing his anxiety.

So how can a mother who feels she needs this kind of clarification of her relationship with her physician bring it about? Let me add here that when any mother in my practice is disgruntled because things aren't going well, be assured that I have been aware of the situation as long as she. I doubt that many doctors are too busy to want to clear the air in an unsatisfactory relationship with a patient. But each person's pride is at stake; and the busier the physician, the less time he has to worry about his side of the bargain. So the responsibility falls to the young mother.

She must appeal to her pediatrician for the particular kind of help she needs. She must offer him enough insight into her situation as a mother to give him the tools to work with her. Of course, she may still lose—she may not be able to motivate him and may feel twice as rejected when she fails. But I doubt that this will happen. For I feel there is nothing more rewarding to a pediatrician than realizing that the parents are working with him as closely and understandingly as he wants to work with them.

So now we come to this question: What can mothers and fathers do to make sure that the relationship with their pediatrician really works?

## *Mothers*

Before you decide on a pediatrician, find out all you can about him or her. First of all, be sure he is competent medically and that he is associated with the hospital you will want to use. (This can be done by calling the hospital or, if there is one, the medical school near you.) If he is on the staff of a good institution, he is very likely to be medically sound.

Try to find a doctor in whom you can have confidence and whose advice you will follow. Nothing is more irritating to a physician who is trying to do his best than to be told how to practice his profession. Constant criticism of his medical decisions is undermining to the doctor's confidence and will be destructive to your relationship.

Further, find out about his personality and his

approach to his patients. Ask other mothers how he runs his practice, how he handles his patients —the adults as well as the children. If he doesn't seem your type, find another doctor.

In my own practice I ask prospective parents to come in to see me before their baby arrives. This prenatal visit accomplishes very little medically, and I do not intend it to. But it lets the mother and father see whether they like me and gives me a chance to see if I like them. Then when any one of us senses that we can't communicate easily and aren't likely to work well together, we still have time to skip out. And by the same token, when we do feel an empathy among us, we can meet again with the new baby—already old friends.

Many of my pediatric friends resent being "looked over," and refer to such parents as "shoppers." I think they are wrong, and feel it is an important step to take before parents and pediatrician adopt each other. In many communities, however, this is not an accepted or possible practice, and a mother who attempts it may endanger her future relationship with a pediatrician. So she must find out what she can about him and then be prepared to work with him.

Once your baby is born and you are making routine visits to the pediatrician, you have an ideal opportunity to solidify your working relationship with him. Weight, measurements, inoculations, feedings, checkups for general health—these are important; but if that were all that needed to be done, any competent paramedical person could see your baby. Indeed, I feel that the essence of such visits is really the exchange of feelings and insights.

Unless a mother lets a part of herself be known, asks questions that really concern her, and reveals to her pediatrician areas where she feels lost, the value of the well-baby visit can certainly be questioned. When a mother and a pediatrician can cement their understanding of each other, when mother and doctor set up a team that can work together for the child's physical *and* psychological well-being, they can face all sorts of crises together. When the crisis is at hand, neither has the time nor energy to worry about the feelings of the other. Hence it is necessary that this be done when the child is well.

I remember the first time I had to cope with an infant in a convulsion at home. In my own anxiety I screamed directions at the mother and father—and they screamed back at me. When the seizure was over and the infant had recovered, we all smiled at how impossible we'd been as a team, all of us frantic together. But we hadn't been ineffective, and we had relied on one another in a marvelous, anxious way to get the child through. And it worked. This kind of teamwork comes about in an emergency, but there *are* easier ways, and parents and doctor should try to be sure they are a team beforehand.


## Fathers

What of a father's role in all this?

Our society has not yet set it up for fathers to participate very much in the delivery of the baby or to stay with the mother and child during the first week in the hospital, and I'm sure we are missing out on an ideal time to get fathers "hooked" on their new infants. But you fathers can feel a part of the whole process if you meet the pediatrician beforehand. Go with your wife when she first sees the new doctor. You can offer her moral support, and you have an ideal opportunity to establish your own relationship with the doctor. Nothing is as flattering to a physician, or as reassuring to him or her about the unity of a family, as the father's participation at an initial visit.

The baby's first checkup visit is also a great time for you to go along. It is a triumph to survive the first, nightmarish month of a new baby, and in no small degree survival depends on your support and effort. Enjoy your part in it!

But even if fathers can be persuaded to go along for the initial meeting with the pediatrician and the first checkup, too often they prefer to stay out of the working side of raising their children—and taking them in for checkups and shots is surely work. At the same time a father may feel that he *should* stay out of his wife's relationship with the child's doctor. Still, paying the bills is not enough.

Perhaps one of the reasons the childrearing literature has neglected fathers is that they have allowed this to happen. Fathers may have a difficult time finding their roles with their children, and a pediatrician who is aware of this can help.

Since many of the fathers in my practice teach or go to school, they are free to come in with their wives at checkup times. When they do, they have a chance to express their own interests in a child's development and voice their own concerns —particularly, I find, about discipline and ways in which they can play a real part in a child's growing up.

I have met over half of "my" fathers, and I am sure we have a better understanding of each other as a result. So when one of them calls me at night or on weekends because his child is ill, we start off with a rapport that otherwise couldn't exist.

There is one other point I would like to make to you fathers. When your child is sick and the pediatrician comes to your house, don't sit in the living room as if you aren't interested. Either go in when he or she looks at the child or ask what you want to know when the examination is over. Show that you are concerned and responsible. Nothing worries doctors so much as an apparent lack of involvement on the father's part.

By this time a father is likely to feel a part of the parent-pediatrician team, and he should feel freer to join his wife on visits when his own concerns deserve it. When the child is ill or when there are mounting tensions at home, when conflict between the parents is contributing to the child's psychological problems, a father should present himself for help to a person who can sort these out with the child's basic interest foremost. If he has already established a good relationship with the pediatrician, he can feel better about turning over this role to him or her.

As a father of adolescent children myself, I need to turn to an objective outsider to pull me out of the scrapes I get into with my children. Our pediatrician can do it. He knows how many of "our" problems are actually my problems, because he has grown to know me over the years. I recommend this to you fathers among my readers.

I would like to see a return to the old days of barter, when one person exchanged his or her work or craft for another's. I would like a father to pay me with his farm produce or his art or his legal advice in exchange for my looking after his child. This would seem an ideal way of directly involving the father by appreciating his role in the child's care. Short of this, getting to know and understand the father's profession and his ways of participating in the family seem vital. A pediatrician should have this opportunity, but he won't make it unless you give him the chance!

## The pediatrician

For several years now, I have been spending part of each day teaching at Harvard Medical School and conducting research with infants. These sides of my profession are very rewarding, both personally and professionally. And I have *learned* to enjoy each of them. But I never had to learn to love the part of each day I spend in my own practice. For twenty years it has been fun and fulfilling.

The horrors of all-night stands by a bedside, of losing a patient I care about, of being awakened at night by so many phone calls that I can't get back to sleep, of answering the same question asked by the same mother month after month, of hearing through the grapevine how I've been criticized by ex-patients—all of these fade away as I drive back from the medical school in Boston across the river to my office in Cambridge, to see a waiting room full of delicious children, of friendly, caring mothers and fathers. I feel like purring the way a young child does when he sees his teddy bear or blanket and heads for it, growling out a low-pitched, excited "There you are!" as he falls upon it.

My family has not had as rewarding a time as I from this profession. Because I love it I work too late and too hard, and there is not enough left of me when I come home. My patients who congratulate my wife on my understanding and kind approach are likely to be greeted with a cold, unbelieving stare. My children have had to compete with many thousands of other children about whom I care and who care about me.

I remember the first "father's day" I attended at my oldest daughter's school. When I sat on the floor next to her as she played, three of my young patients clambered into my lap. My daughter, saddened, turned and walked away to a corner across the room with her back to me. And it was difficult for her to make friends with any of those three classmates for many days afterward.

My children unconsciously emphasize the fact that some of my patients are "their" friends—as if this were incompatible with my relationship with them. And often small children will not come to our house to play without expressing real reluctance; they find it difficult to think of playing in the house of the person who may dole out inoculations and medication. Still, I suspect, my children will profit eventually from the excitement they see in me and the benefits that do sift down to them.

All of us who are doctors have chosen medicine, and especially pediatrics, for our own reasons—we care about working with people and we place great value on the healthy development of children. And although most pediatricians do go through a phase of being convinced that they know more about children and childrearing than parents do, they soon get their comeuppance.

When a young doctor gets out into the "real" world of family medicine, and particularly when he has children of his own, he begins to realize that what *he* thinks is good for the child and what *he* can do to influence the child's development is almost meaningless unless he can effect it through the family, unless he enters into a kind of teamwork and works with the parents for the child.

One young pediatrician said to me the other day, "I guess it's because they're paying me, but I find I'm beginning to like parents!" He is wrong. The payment is only a symbol of what is really happening between them. That doctor is learning the importance and the excitement of forming a working alliance. The feedback from parents who like you and with whom you are effecting results makes pediatrics the most rewarding and exciting profession I know.

I will continue to try to convey the excitement of it to young trainees. And you as parents must do your best to convey the fact that you care to the harried and overworked man you call "your" doctor.

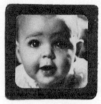 # Helping your child get along with the doctor

No one can expect a child to want to go to the doctor. He or she is full of the same feelings that affect an adult—hating to have to undress in a strange place, hating to be looked at too closely for "what might be wrong," hating to be invaded —by a throat stick, by poking fingers, by a listening device, by eyes that say "we see through you." These feelings do not necessarily mean the child is fearful, but are natural reactions to feelings of privacy and autonomy, natural concerns about whether he is "bad" or "good." No wonder a child dissolves into tears when concerned adults talk seriously about whether his heart murmur is good or bad, or when they remark in passing, "His flat feet are bad, and they are not getting any better." His whole orientation is to be better.

I always shudder in my office when a mother comes in the front door saying, "Alice is going to cry." Alice dutifully picks up her mother's own resistance to coming to my office, and of course she defends herself—by crying. Often I vainly attempt to stop a mother, who, embarrassed by her child's natural tendency to resist my advances in an examination, says, "He won't hurt you!"

This may not have occurred at all to the child, who has simply been protecting himself or herself from my intrusive approaches, but now has a solid and permissible reason for concern. From that moment on, the concern has real substance— he or she should be afraid, because I might hurt. And, of course, I might. But fear need not be at the base of his or her initial reactions. If I have become the child's trusted friend by the time he has to have an inoculation or a blood test, he will trust me when I tell him that this *will* hurt, but not for long, and he may want to cry, of course. And after the hurt is gone, we can be friends again and he can have a reward. After the hurt is over, I remind him that I told him so that he could continue to trust me—for our relationship is too important to endanger it by any lack of honesty or preparation for an unusual hurt.

If parents have a good relationship with the pediatrician, the child is most likely to follow along, and will gradually but surely accept the doctor. In my own practice, I have various ways of helping children to enjoy, rather than dread, their office visits. I feel it is important to me and to them that we have a good relationship. To me and to their parents, it spells the difference between a peaceful and a horrendous visit. But, to them, it means much more. If they can begin to trust a person who will examine, intrude, and even hurt them "for their own good," they are ready for other kinds of relationships—dentists, teachers, shoe clerks, and even other pediatricians. So it is vital to them that we make a "go" with each other. And, for me, a decent relationship offers an entirely new window. I do not feel that my expertise in pediatrics need be confined to a physical evaluation alone. I want very much to understand the child as a person, to see how he reacts to me, to my intrusive exam, to the shots I have to give him. For me, each of these situations is a window into how he copes with stress. With this insight, I can help his parents more, I can see him more fully as a person, and I can let him know that I care about and understand what he is going through in my office.

What is the child going through? He or she is being looked at, invaded, examined, and even hurt. Of course everyone says "it is for your own good," but that just reinforces his resistance, his feeling that he is at fault because he can't understand why all this is important. How could he? I feel that his questions and his fears and his attempts to protect his integrity should be respected. When they are, he can gather self-confidence and a feeling that says, "I'm not bad, I just don't like all this!" And why should he? So I go through a lot of very simple, very inexpensive (in time and money) manipulations to show my respect for these self-protective feelings. And they do work.

Children are given time to play around with toys in the waiting room, and continue their play in the examining room, while we talk. Meanwhile, they are getting familiar with the place. I try to let children make friends with me at their own pace. As they make a few gentle, tentative advances, I return them, but I realize that this takes time. Often I ask mothers to remove their child's clothes gradually as we talk together. With a very frightened child who has no immediate illness or problem, I do only the briefest physical examination, but encourage the mother to bring the child back each week to play on the rocking horses and the slide and to get a lollipop or a balloon. Bit by bit, over a period of time, I begin to wear a stethoscope and the examining procedures are introduced. These weekly visits take only a minute between my regular appointments and after four or five a frightened child generally changes into an eager, cooperative one.

Mothers can help children form a close bond with the doctor by not pushing them or being embarrassed by their resistance in these early visits, and by helping the children feel that this is their *own* doctor. A four-year-old going home after a visit to my office told her mother: *"You* don't know Dr. Brazelton. He's *my* doctor."

There are different stages when the stronger anxiety that interferes begins to peak and shape our relationship:

For the first three or four months the office visits can be calm and happy. At four months the baby is likely to gurgle responsively and even reward me with a smile. But then suddenly at five or six months, the baby discovers that I am a stranger. As long as he or she is seated comfortably in the mother's lap, all is well, but once placed on the examining table and I begin the examination, the infant becomes a wailing terror. If the mother can keep the baby in her lap for as long as possible, and keep her face between the baby's and the doctor, this wailing can at least be delayed. I feel this wailing is in response to my having come *too close.*

At around seven months a baby takes more interest in the office toys, and can be encouraged to accept me. But this relationship breaks down again at about a year. The mother can help the examination along by undressing the child in her lap, and holding him or her while I check ears, nose, throat, and so on. I show how I shall use each instrument by demonstrating it on the mother, "lovey," a toy doll, or even on myself.

In this way the baby can be introduced gradually to each procedure. All of this is done in the mother's safe lap, and I rarely find it too overwhelming for a child of any age. It takes very little extra time for me. When it comes time to examine the belly, measure the head, and weigh the child on the scales, he or she may not like it but has made it through the rest of the exam and is proud. Screeching at this point is almost inevitable.

Setbacks after the booster shot must be counteracted with toys or lollipops and a visit or two without a trauma. As I have said before, parents can help children develop a positive feeling about office visits by making such an extra visit from time to time, just to let the child play in the waiting room with the toys and say hello to me.

From the age of two years, I expect that appointments should become more and more pleasant. At about four or five years of age, there is another brief flurry of resistance (the so-called "oedipal" period). Little girls develop ambivalent feelings about the physical examination. They can become both frightened and overstimulated when I examine their bellies and genital area. If this flurry of excitement can be taken in stride by the parent, and little emphasis put on this part of the visit, the child's ambivalent feelings can be explained to her and they do not intrude on our friendship. Little boys worry, too, but about being hurt. I need to be more understanding and to verbalize some of their fears for them. When I do, they look at me gratefully, and I get the rewarding feeling they are grateful for having these unrecognized feelings brought to light.

When children have had to go to the hospital, or have had an unusually painful experience of any kind, they must be expected to be frightened and worried about its repetition. Their anxiety is not only to be expected—but to be respected. If parents deny it and press them to suppress these feelings, they are urging their children toward a potentially damaging pattern. Denial is an effective defense but it can be a costly one. And I feel that recognition of their residual anxiety is an opportunity for me and for the parents to help children learn to cope more openly with past and future trauma. Hence, when I see them in the hospital or in my office, we talk openly about the event, their feelings and how natural it is for anyone to hate the whole process of being sick, hurt, and separated from home, and to be afraid. Even small children feel guilty about having these feelings and about not being able to handle them "like a good boy (or girl)." I am constantly amazed at the gratitude with which my recognition and acceptance of these feelings is

greeted by small children. After such an event, we
go through the whole process of establishing trust
between us all over again. And in the process I
can work to let them know that I appreciate and
accept them and their reactions. At the same
time, we can agree, often implicitly, that of course
they had to go through it all "for their own good,"
but who likes being hurt—*even* "for their own
good"?

One five-year-old, tousle-haired boy who had
had a necessary tonsillectomy, and had pulled
away from me after that, came into my office for
a "visit"—without trauma or even an exam. As I
told him how sorry I was he'd had to go through
it, and how I knew he must have feelings of anger
and disappointment in me and in his parents for
having let him be hurt, he said, "You didn't even
hurt me yourself, you just *let* me." I realized he
meant that I had let him be hurt. I gathered him
up into my lap, his body stiff and half-resisting, to
say that I was terribly sorry that I had had to "let
him," but I wanted him to feel better than he had,
and to get rid of all those earaches his "tonsils"
had caused. He said then, "But I cried, and I was
sad because I was bad." When we talked about
how natural it was for him to cry because he was
hurt, and that it wasn't bad, nor was he bad, he
began to relax in my lap. Eventually he
brightened and said, "You tell me it's okay to cry
when I get a shot here, don't you?"
Enthusiastically, I nodded. He said, "But I didn't
like all that hospital stuff." I realized that he had
been pressing himself to like it because he had
taken our words seriously, that "it was for his own
good." When I could say to him that *no one* liked

all that hospital stuff, even if it was for their own good, he laughed out loud, with relief. We were friends again, and our mutual trust secure.

As children get older, it becomes more and more important to see that they have time alone with their pediatrician, to encourage them to speak directly about themselves. At about the time of preadolescence, the parent should make a point of remaining in the waiting room, while the child goes in to see the doctor alone. In this way, as they become adolescents, children can come to think of the pediatrician as someone whom they can contact themselves, when they have questions which they find hard to ask parents. A lifelong habit of responsibility about one's own health, of taking the initiative and seeing a doctor before serious illness strikes can be fostered in these adolescent years. A relationship which has gradually developed between doctor and patient can really pay off in the adolescent years. I have had many adolescents who "just come by"—to ask me about the relative merits of the "pill" or of hard drugs—at a time when I am pretty sure that they have few outlets for their questions except their peers—who are as confused as they.

The opportunities for establishing and valuing a relationship between doctor and child make pediatrics an exciting field. To become a member of the child's team as he struggles to deal with our world is a priceless opportunity.

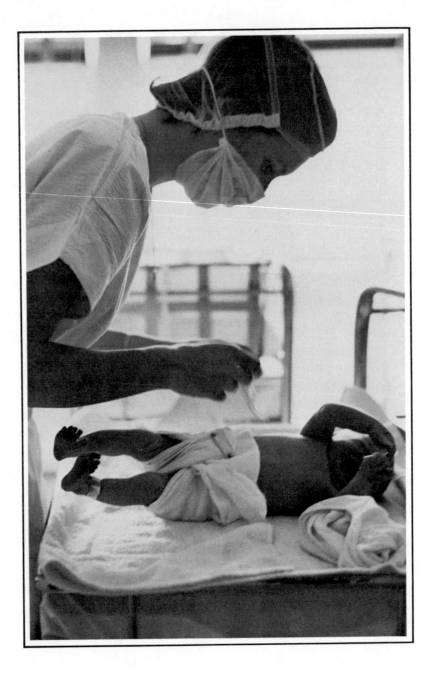

## Chapter 2

# What childbirth drugs can do to your child

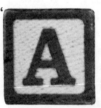"re you sure that's my baby?"

"He's too sleepy to nurse. Are you positive there's nothing wrong with him?"

"Why can't she stay awake? Did I do something to her in labor?"

These queries, familiar to any pediatrician, reflect the fears of damage and imperfection that all mothers have about a newborn baby. But for mothers who have been awake, actively participating in the delivery, the impact of these fears seems to be softened. On the other hand, when a mother has been drugged and made oblivious to the birth, the drowsy, unresponsive infant compounds her anxiety.

I am concerned about the routine use of drugs during childbirth, concerned about the subtle ways these drugs often affect the earliest experiences of the mother and her newborn infant. This concern is highlighted for me by an incident that occurred a few years ago while I was in Mexico doing research.

In a remote southern village I witnessed the delivery of a young girl's first baby. All during her pregnancy she had led an entirely routine existence, working from dawn to dusk. Her husband and his family, with whom they lived, saved extra eggs and bits of meat for her because she was with child, but she was spared no physical work in the day-to-day life in the compound.

As she went into labor, her own mother and sisters with their families—children and dogs included—as well as all the members of her husband's family assembled in the largest hut of the compound. A toothless old midwife was summoned and given the role of "conducting" the delivery. And indeed she became the conductor of a large, supportive symphony orchestra.

While the girl knelt with her head in her mother's lap, her husband stood behind her, tightening a cinch around her waist at each labor pain. This served to put pressure on the fundus of the uterus, thus helping to ease the pain and adding gentle pressure to push out the infant. As the girl groaned and cried with each contraction, every member of the group—there were twenty or thirty—groaned with her in rising, keening wails. When she became silent and wept between contractions, they listened respectfully, assuring her that all women had to bear this labor, this work, and that all survived its burden. The girl alternately whimpered and cursed, blaming her husband, her mother, the gods, for her plight. All the family nodded with understanding, and the old midwife chanted magical charms. Chickens and dogs wandered in and out of the hut. Children raced around the seated relatives; young babies were nursed by their own new mothers.

As the girl's pains intensified so did the excitement in the hut. A great deal of grain alcohol (called *posh*) was being consumed, especially by the midwife, who for some reason or other announced that she was leaving. With the midwife's departure all the supportive keening stopped, and soon afterward the girl's labor came to a complete halt. The women shook their heads sadly.

"The baby's stuck, and the mother and the baby will die," they said ominously.

I was horrified at this failure of confidence and support, and I begged them to keep their fears to themselves.

"She knows it," they said.

And indeed her weeping had reached a peak. I urged her to get up off her knees and walk around vigorously, assuring her that this kind of exercise helped reinstitute labor. I also suggested that she lie on her back and push with her legs spread apart. To please me she followed my suggestions, but halfheartedly, and the women nodded knowingly when the maneuvers failed.

After two anxious hours, the men in the hut sent out a large bottle of liquor to secure the services of a new, older, wiser, more toothless midwife. As she walked into the hut, she ordered everyone to his post—the men to gathering wood; the women to boiling water, washing baby clothes, cooking *tortillas.* She shook the girl's pelvis and announced

confidently, "Now she's unstuck," told the husband
to start pulling on the cinch again and began to
chant loudly. In minutes, labor started and the
keening resumed. Within an hour, to the delighted
crescendo of supporting relatives, she delivered a
healthy, active, alert infant.

There is no need to romanticize this birth or to
issue a clarion call of "back to the midwife" and
"down with all drugs during childbirth." I don't
know what the maternal and infant death rates are
in that village. I am sure they are higher than in
our good hospitals—but maybe not higher than in
our poor ones. I do know that this birth in Mexico
was for me a stunning revelation of the many
things we have lost in our drug-prone society.

The marvelous support of the extended family,
the understanding of the women for the girl's pain
and fears, the importance of a leading figure such
as the midwife, who has the knowledge, the
authority—and, yes, the magic—to conduct a
ceremony that partakes of the sacred—all somehow
are used in the service of a natural event. Giving
birth is a normal life process of a healthy woman,
and the excitement and joy of it ultimately
outweigh the pain and anxiety.

In our medicated society we have eradicated
some of the pain and anxiety, but I'm afraid we
have eradicated more of the excitement and joy.
Pregnancy, labor, and delivery are thought of as
essentially a disease in the United States. As a
result the anxiety and fear and pain are medically
treated as if they were evil and destructive
symptoms of the "condition" rather than positive
forces that mobilize a woman for an awesome,

prodigious, and usually enormously rewarding experience—the birth of a child.

I do not presume to say that all women can or should have their babies without medication and medical sophistication. When that Mexican baby was "stuck," I fervently wished that we were in a hospital rather than in a hut and that I were an obstetrician rather than a pediatrician. But I do feel that in obstetrics, as in many branches of medicine, we may have gone too far in our zeal to "treat" rather than to understand and help.

The reasons for our medicated approach to birth are many—and many of them are well-founded. I remember one woman who was determined to go through labor without medication or anesthetic. She stood by the side of her bed, gritting her teeth, holding on to the guardrail, all her sphincters as tight as she was, saying, "I want the baby to come. I want the baby to come." She was the picture of ambivalence. Of course she wanted to deliver, but her tense body was responding to the anxiety she felt and the result was a difficult twenty-four-hour labor. As soon as she was medicated, however, her tension dissolved and she delivered the baby in short order.

I am sure that such "needless suffering" weighs heavily on any obstetrician, and there are many instances like this one in which medication is necessary, or at least extremely useful. I must also add that I realize obstetrics is a complex, sophisticated member of the medical specialties. Finally I want to make clear that I do not presume to know about or see the whole obstetrics picture. My remarks must be seen in the light of my

prejudice about the product of delivery. I am
frankly pro-baby. And I do not like what drugs
administered to a woman in labor do to her baby.
If this seems to set up a mother-versus-baby
conflict of interest, let me hasten to say that what
troubles me most is that drugs can rob mother and
child alike of important experiences in the first
weeks of their life together.

Many of the drugs used to make labor easier and
less painful for the mother affect the baby's
adjustment to his or her new world. Although they
do not have permanent impact on the newborn or
on the brain and cannot, in that sense, be
considered "dangerous," we are finding more and
more evidence that the medicated prelude to birth
is not so simple for the baby as doctors had
assumed.

Traditionally obstetricians have been responsible
for the care of the infant in the delivery room, and
only in cases of trouble was the pediatrician
summoned. For the past decade, however,
pediatricians have been monitoring the newborn,
using tests that reflect his or her adjustment to the
immediate change-over from a parasitic existence
in the uterus to an extrauterine independence.

The Apgar score, named for its originator, Dr.
Virginia Apgar, an anesthesiologist at Columbia
University, is administered at one, five, and fifteen
minutes after delivery. It grades the baby on five
behavioral responses: (1) his color (from deep blue
to pink); (2) his efforts to breathe (from slow and
labored to fast and jerky to regular and easy); (3)
his sucking response when he is offered a gloved
finger; (4) his general muscle tone (from limp to

active and resistant) when his legs and arms are moved; (5) his irritability when his nose is stroked gently with a light object (he should sneeze or wiggle his face).

After these tests are administered, the baby is injected as a matter of routine with vitamin K to prevent bleeding and has silver nitrate solution dropped into his eyes to protect him from any maternal vaginal infection. He is wrapped warmly, and tilted head down in bed so that gravity can drain out the mucus and fluid that has filled his airways and lungs in the uterus.

While in the delivery room every baby goes through an initial stage of alertness. Usually his energies have been mobilized by his mother's labor; but even without labor, as is the case in cesarean delivery, he is stimulated by the noisy, cold, and light world suddenly confronting him. The baby responds to labor, to birth, and to this new environment with all his emergency resources. The Apgar score, given before the newborn is injected and swaddled, reflects his best efforts. It has become the standard method of "evaluating" the newborn. Two points each are given for optimal responses; most infants score nine or ten. A score below six is thought to be a warning of possible trouble.

Since about 90 percent of babies have an Apgar score of seven or over, doctors have developed a certain smugness about the treatment of newborns. The high number of adequate scores has reassured most obstetricians that they need not question the routine practices of premedication and anesthetics.

Eight years ago, however, I was perplexed by

many of the babies I saw in the nurseries of our lying-in hospitals. Each one had been sent from the delivery room with an excellent Apgar score. They arrived in the nurseries thirty minutes after delivery, were stimulated by the nurses with a bath and clean clothes, swaddled again, and placed head tilted down in their cribs.

But all too often, as the nursery nurse made one of her frequent checks, she found the new infant blue, cold, breathing shallowly, and difficult to rouse. When she tried to awaken him, he choked up mucus, coughed halfheartedly, and made very little effort to rid himself of it.

Since new infants are equipped with a magnificently effective gag response that makes it nearly impossible for them to choke, this lethargy was even more striking. The nurse helped him to breathe by clapping him vigorously on the back, but when she stopped, he fell quickly back into his listless, unresponsive state. Although doctors and nurses are used to this kind of setback, it is still very disturbing.

We have observed that after the infant's high-key response to the birth process, exhaustion sets in. After a normal, nonmedicated delivery, infants are alternately sleepy and overexcited, disorganized and difficult to reach for twenty-four to forty-eight hours. What I learned from watching these "high score" babies, however, was that when the mother has been medicated, there is a lengthening of the baby's depressed period; it can continue for a week after delivery, rather than for two days.

We know that the medication given to a mother

immediately before delivery passes through the placenta to her baby. If she has a perceptible level of depressant drugs circulating in her system when the umbilical cord is cut, so has the baby. The mother can wear hers off in a matter of hours, since her liver and kidneys are functioning at full adult tilt and will detoxify the drug. Not so with her infant. His liver is taken up with the job of breaking down extra blood cells and eliminating the jaundice all new babies pile up in the first few days, so that it cannot deal with the drugs immediately. His immature kidneys don't excrete depressant drugs very well. And his immature brain stores them for *at least* a week after birth, concentrating them around the midbrain, which is responsible for much of his behavior. No wonder he is relatively dopey for a week or two after delivery! The real wonder is how he functions at all.

Because of my keen interest in establishing a solid start for the mother and her infant, I am very disturbed when I see a new mother saddled with a very sleepy baby for his first, crucial week of their life together. *All* mothers have deep fears about a newborn baby. And *all* mothers are upset by the exhausted baby they see a day or so after birth. I reassure them that the depressed period will pass, and it does—but for many mothers and babies, not quickly enough. Partly because the baby is too sleepy to nurse at the breast and partly because his poor sucking does not adequately stimulate her breasts, the mother never produces an adequate milk supply during this period. Even more disturbing to me, however, is the emotional effect that such a depressed baby must have on an eager new mother.

The noted naturalist Konrad Lorenz has observed the "imprinting" process among animals. He made proper "mother goose" noises to goslings as they first hatched and found that thereafter they followed him about as if he were their mother. The British psychiatrist John Bowlby has recently pointed out that there is an imprinting process for human babies too that must take place if a firm, positive mother-infant relationship is to be established. The many gentle and loving acts a mother instinctively performs undoubtedly set off the complex responses the new baby shows to her —the brightening, softening look that comes over the infant's face as his mother speaks gently to him; the way the squirming, stiff infant begins to cuddle into her arms as she rocks him; the way he turns first his eyes, then his whole head, to her soft voice; the way his eyes blink sleepily and gradually open; and finally after wandering about dazedly, the way each eye separately fixes on her face and awareness seems to dawn, accompanied by an alerting of all of his features, a new shine in his eyes and a quieting of the rest of his body.

These are *not* figments of a mother's imagination or her wishful dreaming. They are evidence of the complex responses with which we are just beginning to credit newborns, and which need appropriate triggers from the mother.

But a new mother needs appropriate triggers too! She is just as disintegrated, just as uncerebral as her new infant—rendered so by her recent

experience in labor and delivery and reinforced by
her anxiety to be a good mother.

Watch any new mother as she fumbles over her
new baby—as she tries one technique after another
to get him to suck, to bubble him, to stop his legs
from thrashing about long enough to get the diaper
pinned without pinning him to the diaper! She is
floundering just as he is. Nothing can bind her to
this wiggly creature as effectively as his rewarding
response when she happens upon the correct
method. She needs his response every bit as much
as he needs hers.

What happens, then, to a woman's mothering
responses when she meets a doped, listless,
seven-pound thing? Can she maintain the high
peak of excitement, the initial level of investment?

I am sure there are many women who can
muster greater maternal energy when faced with
an unresponsive baby who, they can rationalize,
"needs" them even more than a sprightly one. But
is this a proper start for a baby who will not
eventually need an overprotective environment?

I compared the breast-feeding responses of
babies whose mothers had received the average
doses of barbiturates two to eight hours before
delivery, those who had had an inhalant anesthetic
administered during the actual delivery, and those
who had received no medication at all. The babies
of nonmedicated mothers recovered quickly from
the birth experience, and by the third day they
were able to nurse and were beginning to gain
weight. Babies born with the aid of a spinal,
caudal, or an inhalant anesthetic seemed to suffer
only minor effects and also recovered rapidly. But

babies delivered with barbiturate premedicants
had weight gain delayed by twenty-four to
forty-eight hours and had impaired responses to
the nursing situation. I wondered how an
inexperienced mother must react to this
unresponsiveness and lag in weight gain. Of
course, I felt that the lag was due not only to the
baby's dulled responses but also to the
physiological effect of depressant medications on
the mother. (See chart.)

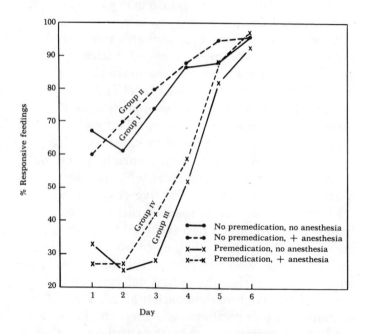

I would like to urge a more considered approach
to "routine" medication and anesthetics. Let these
drugs be used when necessary—but as the

exception, not the rule. The mother who must be medicated should be told of the problems the drugs may cause, and the obstetrician should help her and her infant adjust afterward.

The woman whose goal is an unmedicated delivery should discuss this with her obstetrician, preferably at her first visit, so that she may learn how he feels about the use of drugs. Although there are a few obstetricians today who are not willing to accept a woman's preferences, most are eager to oblige a woman who is, in effect, promising to help in the delivery of her baby. The obstetrician should support her through her labor and reassure her if she reaches a point where she and the baby will profit by medication. Even if she cannot—or should not—hold out for the entire labor, the longer she can wait, the less effect any necessary medication will have.

Thanks to such groups as the International Childbirth Education Association, who teach France's Lamaze method and England's Grantly Dick Read system, childbirth without drugs is staging a comeback. These groups, which have mushroomed throughout the country, have forced hospitals and physicians to accept unmedicated, nonanesthetized deliveries. They also have been responsible for the creation and training of "nurse supports," who teach women what to expect in labor and delivery and how to cope with it. The groups also have urged that the husband learn the signals and signs of labor's progress so that he can participate actively in his wife's experience and can be a strong, constant support for her. What a superb answer to the gap that was left when we forswore the ways of our "primitive" ancestors and became "civilized"—and overmedicated!

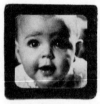

# Education for childbirth

The preceding article was written several years ago in an attempt to reinforce an already swelling movement led by the International Childbirth Education Association. Their efforts to provide women in the United States with choices about whether or not to use anesthesia for their delivery began in Boston in 1956, and I was very interested in their ideas. At that time, the maternity hospitals were still using a great deal of medication to sedate mothers, so that their labor pains were minimal, and childbirth could be forgotten thereafter. But we pediatricians had just begun to be aware of the fact that the infants were sedated and limp for as much as ten days after delivery. I was also pretty sure that mothers' postpartum blues were worsened by the aftereffects on them of the medication used for delivery. And in a study of a group of breast-fed babies, we found that the ones whose mothers had no medication recovered and began to gain weight twenty-four to forty-eight hours before the group of infants belonging to medicated mothers. This implied to me that the mothers' milk production was cut down while the medication was affecting

her, and the mother-child unit was bound to be
slowed down in their initial takeoff. At this point,
I realized that U.S. medicine was treating labor
and delivery as if it were a pathological condition,
a disease, and *not* a great event, a turning point
for a young couple. What a brainwashing this was
for young parents who wanted to get off to a good
start with their new babies. If everyone treated
the act of childbirth as if it were something to be
avoided or gotten through, the joy of becoming
parents was already seriously undermined. And
instead of a triumphant achievement, it becomes
something to be afraid of. This impressed me as a
very serious error on our part as physicians. If we
reinforce the anxieties parents already have, by
adding our own to them, we have only made it
more likely that women will indeed need
medication and sedatives—to allay this very
anxiety.

The childbirth education groups began to
educate pregnant women about their role in labor,
about ways to alleviate pain for themselves, and
they made it possible for many women to be
successful in mastering labor without painkillers.

Now they have gone on to press young fathers
into service. They are being educated as to what
to expect, how to support their wives, and when to
call in the professionals. This is another big step
in reinforcing the strengths and joy with which
young prospective parents come to their new
roles. Fathers who have been through this
experience are absolutely hooked on the baby, and
eager to support their wives in the new family
unit. So I am all for the growing trend to offer

people the opportunity and the professional
back-up to make their own choices about this
important event in their lives.

Not every young mother could or should go
through labor without sedatives or analgesics. I
cited an example in this chapter of an extreme
instance. And I think there are many, many
couples who would be more stressed than elated
by the experience. I do *not* recommend natural
childbirth to them, nor do I feel that they should
feel guilty about not being able to go through with
it. My main goal is for each couple to be able to
make his and her choice, without unnecessary
interference from the medical profession. If there
are open choices, and the participants all
recognize them, then when the obstetrician must
decide to use medication, both the parents and he
or she will know the decision was based on expert
medical judgment.

The value of preparing all couples for labor and
childbirth, even if they do not plan to go through
with natural childbirth, is very great. First of all,
preparation alleviates much of the fear of
delivering a baby, or it puts it in proper
perspective. Then, a young woman can hold off
medication for a longer period, and the
cumulative effect on the baby is minimized.
Knowledge of delivery for her and for her
husband may seem frightening before preparation
is under way, but I have never found that parents
feel it is anything but supportive and
anxiety-relieving. Participation in preparatory
courses must be very reassuring in another way—
pregnant women (and their husbands) get to know

each other and to realize that they are not the
only ones who are facing this challenge.

So, I am a strong advocate of education before
delivery, as well as of education for parenthood. It
is a big adjustment. It has to be if you really care.
Becoming a mother or a father, giving up one's
girlhood and boyhood adolescence to take on a
new, responsible role, becomes more frightening
the more you care. But the rewards can be equal
to the frustrations and to the work of making this
adjustment. Having a fascinating, responsive,
rewarding baby can be one of the most thrilling
experiences one will ever have. And if you can
consciously participate in the event, can master it
for yourself, however much or little, the event can
become a real turning point for you—and a
cornerstone of your future family.

Of course from the baby's standpoint, the sooner
you can be awake and available, the better it's
likely to be for him. In a study done in Cleveland
by Drs. Marshall Klaus and John Kennell, both
pediatricians, mothers (and later, fathers) were
given the chance to get used to their premature
infants while they were still in the premature
nurseries. Until that time, parents of premature
babies had been forced to stand behind glass
panes to look at their children. All of them
reported that this protective glass and the
enforced separation made them feel hopelessly
inadequate for their tiny infants—and even
strengthened a feeling they'd already had, that
they had done something wrong which had
resulted in their babies being premature in the
first place. By the time these parents got a chance

to take their infants home, they were thoroughly frightened, and felt helpless for several months in the effort of getting to know the babies as people.

Drs. Klaus and Kennell brought new parents into the premature nursery, urged them to reach into the incubators to touch their babies, then to hold them, and finally to feed them. Since this was pretty frightening at first, the nursery nurses stood by and taught the new parents how to handle and feed their premature infants. By the time they could take their babies home, the parents knew them, they had fed and changed them, and they were able to cuddle and hold them with love rather than fear. The infants did nearly twice as well as the untouched babies—gained weight, began to develop more quickly, and at a year, both parents and babies still showed the significant effect of having been encouraged to be together from the first. I think this kind of approach can help normal babies also. The sooner we can unite a new family, and can support them, *under* the protection of hospital personnel, as they get to know each other, the more effective will be our efforts to get the family off to a good start. Not only do they feel closer before they must face it alone, but they also feel that there is someone in the medical profession who cares about them as a family, and they may even be able to turn back for help more quickly when they need it.

Rooming in with the new baby is a step in this direction, and all of the experience with it has been basically good. I think there are real drawbacks to it, however. All mothers need a chance to recover from labor and delivery *before*

they take on the responsibility for the new infant.
New mothers must regain their physical strength,
and a new baby is demanding and dependent.
Mothers with other children at home need rest
before they reassume the responsibility for the
family. But after they have recovered, most
mothers should have the new baby near them in
the hospital for at least a full day, to learn his or
her rhythms and sleep-cry patterns. This can be a
real opportunity for each to get to know the other
—baby, mother, father—in the protected isolation
of the hospital. It can be a real investment in the
future of the family.

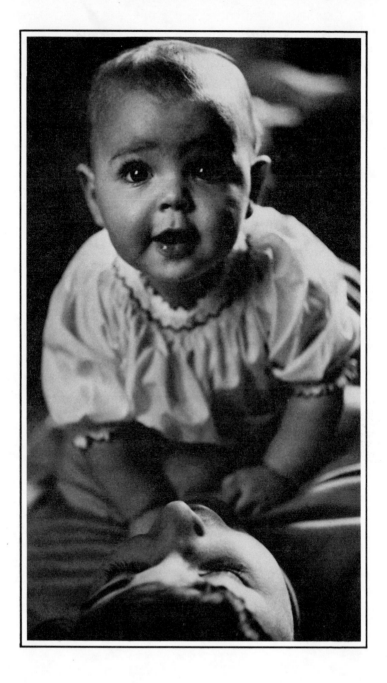

## Chapter 3

# Trial by motherhood: the first-time blues

"The big moment had finally arrived. My baby was all mine. My husband and I were to be together again; we were a real family at last!"

As Mrs. Clay sat in my office she began to talk about becoming a mother for the first time—the climax of nine long months of waiting for the reality of a baby, of enduring and even enjoying the pain and anguish of delivering him and of experiencing the mixture of euphoria and uneasiness that comes with the inevitable changes that follow childbirth.

"I was so relieved that the delivery was over and that we were all right. Of course I'd worried about myself and whether I'd make it, but my main fears had been about the baby—would he be okay? Had I done something in pregnancy that might have damaged him? Would I be able to love him? Then when I saw how perfect he was, when

I held him and nursed him, I became giddy with relief and pleasure. I saw everyone, including Bob, my husband, through a sort of pink glow.

"I remember feeling very comforted by the fact that there were people in charge of me and my baby. Knowing that allowed me to lie back and enjoy Mark as much as I did, because underneath I was also frightened.

"I couldn't and still can't visualize myself as a mother. If I let myself think about it, I get goose bumps all over. I look at Mark in his sleep and think, You poor little helpless, motherless thing. Then he wakes up. He looks at me, and his face brightens as I pick him up. He nestles in my arms and turns his searching, rooting mouth toward my breast. My shivers disappear, and I settle down into the most disgusting puddle of sloppy, sentimental well-being."

Mrs. Clay nestled into the chair as she talked. When she came into my office she had been stiff and tense. Mark had sensed his mother's tension and awakened to cry. She had rocked him awkwardly. Then as she became more relaxed, her behavior became gentler, smoother, and much more soothing, and Mark was once more asleep in her arms.

Though she had been telling me about the big adjustment she had had to make after Mark was born and how hard it had been, her composure now showed me that it had been successful. She was already a mother—a person who had made it with herself and with her new baby. This is a big step for any woman with her first child, and one that most women doubt they'll be able to make.

And it is not a development that necessarily comes quickly and easily.

As Mrs. Clay recalled her experiences in the first weeks after taking Mark home from the hospital, her eyes grew moist. She explained the tears by saying, "I had a picture in my mind of my husband and myself as the handsome young couple we had always been. Now there was Mark too, and we would be a picture-book family. It never occurred to me that this was only one of the pictures we'd fit into, and that there were others a lot more realistic and more representative of what becoming a family really is!

"Those first weeks at home were like a nightmare. You're too tired and depressed in the beginning to be able to separate what is really happening from what you imagine may be happening. At the beginning I felt like crying or screaming most of the time. If Bob hadn't been so understanding and patient . . . if my mother hadn't come over to help at just the crucial moments . . . if Mark hadn't been so good . . . I *know* I would have cracked, I felt so inadequate as a mother. But each week was easier than the last, and now that he's four weeks old, I'm even sure we're going to make it."

The kind of feelings that Mrs. Clay described to me are related to the depression that comes in the postpartum period. This depression is universal— all new mothers experience it—and its causes are partly physical, partly psychological.

The physical part is due to the tremendous reorganization a woman's body must go through after the delivery of a baby and the inordinate amount of energy she must expend to recover. Of course she is making a big psychological adjustment too, and this also makes demands on her. In our society, where members of families live far apart and where a young mother is expected to "make it" with very little physical or psychological support from outside, it becomes even harder.

In most cultures there are extended families hovering about a new mother. In the Mayan culture in Central America, for example, the new mother is wrapped up with her swaddled baby for several weeks while the women of her extended family allow her to regress to a kind of infancy of her own as she adjusts to her baby. In some parts of Africa a new mother is brought food for her household, her house is kept clean by relatives, and she is expected to spend all her time recovering and learning to "know herself as a mother."

In our own modern society there is a built-in loneliness for the new mother and an expectation of independence during this critical time, which certainly adds to the pressures. Not only have most young couples moved away from their family homes physically, but also they try to free themselves of feelings of dependency on parents by attempting to deny any value in the ways of older people.

Of course, a young mother and father who do "make it alone" in this struggle to care for and cope with a new and dependent human being are rewarded with all the glowing excitement of meeting a new responsibility successfully, and their rewards are enhanced with every new step in the infant's development.

Though the satisfactions are obvious, as a pediatrician I feel it is important for new parents to be aware of the often undiscussed side of this adjustment, for in my experience *all* new parents go through the same kinds of desperate emotional struggle. Because they feel inadequate as parents, they are angry with the baby, with their spouse, their families, and especially with themselves. So I hope that by learning of Mrs. Clay's story, other new parents, particularly new mothers, will gain the assurance that they aren't unique or alone in feeling beset.

Mrs. Clay described her feelings as she left the hospital with her husband and baby. "When we settled into the car and the nurse handed Mark over to me, I had that 'complete family' sense and felt elated. But not for long. Because we'd barely started the car when Mark began to cry. As he built up to a screaming fit, Bob began to get jumpy, and he nearly crashed through an intersection. I bounced Mark, frantically changed his position, wondered how I could feed him or change him in the car and got more and more desperate. As he cried I began to cry too.

"Bob was so upset that he pulled over to the side of the street. Not knowing which one of us to comfort first, he fumbled alternately at Mark's clothes and at me. I think he intended to help me get a breast uncovered to feed Mark, but his efforts were so clumsy and ineffectual that he made me laugh. That relieved the tension and we all relaxed.

"At home my mother was waiting. I'd told her I
wanted just the three of us to step across the
threshold as a family, but she had ignored my
request that she not be there. A lucky thing too,
because by the time I'd struggled up the three
flights of stairs to our apartment—stitches aching
at every step, muscles I'd never dreamed of
screaming at me—and by the time Bob had
brought Mark up, wriggling out of all his
swaddling blankets, I'd *had it!*

"It was pure joy to have Mother take Mark and
change him, pat me into a chair, and hand me a
clean, quiet baby to feed. After he had nursed,
Mother changed Mark again, and we put him into
his crib in the corner of our room. I fell on my
bed laughing at Bob, who was now trying to show
me the results of his nest-building efforts while I
was away. At this point Mother sensed that it was
time to go, and we gratefully let her out.

"The next few days were like a kaleidoscope of
overreactions. There were tears from me,
fumbling help from Bob, unforeseen crises that
were magnified out of all proportion, and Mark
sailing through it all."

In the hope that it will help other young
mothers to see how universal their problems are, I
asked Mrs. Clay to describe some of the stages she
went through.

*His first night at home:* "I hardly slept at all.
Although I'd roomed in with him in the hospital
for two days, the nurses had taken him away
for an eight-hour stretch out of every twenty-four
so that I could get some rest. Maybe that was
the reason for some of my anxiety, since I'd

never spent a whole day and night with him.

"I fed him at ten P.M. as I had at the hospital. By midnight I was sitting up in bed, waiting for him to cry. By two o'clock I was hovering over him. By three, when he finally stirred, I literally grabbed him out of bed to feed him.

"I'm sure he knew how tense I was, because he never really settled down to eat. He fussed and whimpered for an hour. I kept trying to push a nipple into his mouth. He twisted and turned, shutting his mouth tight to reject it. The more he fussed, the harder I tried. We were rapidly building up to an impasse.

"Then Bob took him into the other room to rock him and brought back to me a calm, ready baby. After a relatively peaceful feeding, I handed him back to Bob to change while I edged off to bed. I finally slept from five to six thirty."

*His first day at home:* "One would think it was all worry and no fun. Not at all. That first day at home was the greatest I've ever spent. As we made it through the first day, the three of us on our own, I felt as I had when I was learning to ride a bike. I got that same giddy, excited feeling of 'It's me that's doing this!'

"Mark was great. He took his feedings well. He even seemed to be getting to know me. When I came up to his crib, he stopped fussing to listen to me and to wait for me to pick him up. I even thought he smiled at me, but that, everyone says, was wishful thinking."

*Daily crying periods:* "Toward the end of the first week, Mark became fussier. It was as if he had sensed in the beginning that I couldn't have

stood his being difficult. Of course, I understood
that he was still quiet and dopey after the struggle
of being born. Whatever it was, that period of just
waking and sleeping for the first few days was a
blessing. Many of my friends have told me that
their babies were upset and disorganized at first.
I'm not sure how I'd have managed if he had been
as disorganized as I was.

"When he did begin to develop a 'fussy period'
each day, I wasn't ready for it. Although he slept
and ate well, he began to wake up every afternoon
to fuss. This was just about the time Bob was
expected home, so I tried hard to quiet Mark. I
wanted Bob to see how well Mark was doing. But
the harder I tried, the more difficult Mark
became.

"I tried everything—swaddling him, a pacifier,
an extra feeding, carrying him and bouncing him
—but he kept crying. And my attempts to soothe
him just seemed to add fuel to his crying. I
blamed myself, thinking, I'm hopeless as a
mother! Or I began to cast about for reasons: Was
he hungry? cold? wet? Did he have colic? Did he
need more sucking? Was he getting enough love?

"Then I learned that most babies need a fussy
period at the end of the day—to let off steam, for
exercise, or for reasons of their own—and that if
it came at regular times and the baby was gaining
and doing well otherwise, I could relax. Since
then I've been able to let him fuss for a period of
fifteen to twenty minutes at a stretch. I give him
sugar water to get up the bubble he's cried down
and then put him back to cry it out some more.
Now I think Mark and I are much happier with

each other. He's relieved to be left alone at times.
I'm relieved that his fussing is not all my fault."

Making too much over the baby's fussiness and
too much in the way of anxious attempts to keep
him quiet lead to a tenser infant who cries even
harder. Most of this fussing stops when the baby
is about ten weeks old, when he can do other
things to let off steam—such as gurgle, laugh, or
watch his hands move.

As the baby grows and becomes more sociable,
he will use this same regular "fussing time" to be
his most communicative with the family. This
makes me believe that the earlier periods may
represent his first, ineffectual attempts to reach
out to the world around him. With time and
maturity, he finds more successful ways of
reaching out.

*Feeding problems:* "Although I seemed to
produce enough milk for Mark in the hospital, I
found it much harder to keep it coming after I got
home. The anxiety I had about him, the tension I
lived with as we adjusted to each other, my
restless activity, all seemed to cut down on my
milk supply. Fortunately I had been in contact
with La Leche League, an organization that
promotes the nursing of babies, and I had their
literature to guide me. By resting more and
drinking liquids frequently, and by letting Mark
nurse more frequently in the bad periods, my
milk quickly built back up."

Resting and drinking liquids are important
factors in building up the new mother's milk
supply. It is also a good idea to limit visitors
drastically during the first few days—both to

protect the baby from infection and to give the mother a chance to shore up her energies. Mrs. Clay told me that during those early days "every visitor demanded a kind of energy from me, and that interfered with my big job—that of producing milk for Mark." After the first week, however, her milk became more established.

"I noticed at least twice that Mark's hunger and my milk supply were out of balance with each other. In one case he needed more frequent feedings than I could give him. In the other I suddenly realized he wasn't taking enough from me at each feeding, and I was getting overloaded and uncomfortable as a result. Now we are sailing along—in balance—and I think I can handle it."

In explaining the importance of this balance to Mrs. Clay, I pointed out that a baby's development and his physical needs for food do not increase on a smoothly ascending slope. More likely the baby takes a growth spurt, holds it for a period, and then spurts again. At such times he may get ahead of his mother's milk supply, which is increasing more smoothly and continuously. But by more frequent demands for milk from his mother, he brings her supply up to his need.

Sometimes the baby may push her too hard, in which case the milk supply may get ahead of him. Then the mother must push the child to keep up with her. The most wonderful thing about breast feeding is the interaction and responsiveness between mother and child.

Although I believe breast feeding is better than bottle feeding, I am not extreme in my attitudes. If the need exists, I never hesitate to urge a mother to use an "emergency" formula once or twice a day. If a mother continues to rest and drink fluids to build up her milk—and is determined to nurse—the formula can be a good crutch. But the young mother must be careful not to feel inadequate just because she gives the baby a bottle or two each day—such feelings can wreck the nursing effort.

The best situation is when the mother is sufficiently relaxed to use an occasional bottle for no other reason than that it gives her a rest. After all, it is important for a new mother to feel she can get away for a few hours—to go out with her husband for a restorative fling or to buy herself something as a "pick-me-up."

*Play periods:* "At first I felt like putting Mark to bed as soon as I'd fed him. I was so afraid of hurting him or of not knowing what to do with him if he got too stimulated. Somewhere along the way I realized that he seldom went straight to sleep after eating; he lay awake in bed, looking around. Sometimes he would be fussy until I picked him up again. Then he would quiet down, brighten, and just stare at me. If I rocked him, he looked peaceful and happy.

"Now that he's a little older, if I tickle him or talk softly to him, he smiles or opens his eyes wide to watch me. He follows the movements of a mobile I set up above his crib. When it goes too fast, he just shuts his eyes and turns away. I also notice he does that if I talk loudly or if I try too hard to make him smile. He turns me off by turning his head away or half closing his eyes in a dull look.

"If I prop him up, I notice he is already trying to hold his body and head upright. His eyes get wider open as he sits there, taking everything in. It's when I hold him on my shoulder that he is at his most alert. He looks all around the room. When I put him on his belly, he makes crawling motions and even pushes himself across the bed. He lifts his head up to look around and then plops it down on one side or the other. Then he will bring his fist up to suck on it while he lies there on his belly.

"He seems to enjoy his father too. Bob already treats him 'like a boy.' This means that he can throw the baby up into the air and catch him or make him do vigorous exercises. I have asked Bob why he feels this kind of play is just for boys. His answer is, 'You wouldn't understand.' Men are such chauvinists!"

Mrs. Clay is right. From the very first, men treat little boys differently from little girls. This is not necessarily because of any "male" characteristics that are built into the baby, but more likely because of an expectation the father has. Mothers act differently with boys too, but this is often so unconscious that I'm sure it would be hard to make them aware of the differences in their behavior.

From recent research, though, it does appear that newborn girl babies are a bit different from boys. They are more watchful and will look around for longer periods. Boy babies, on the other hand, are physically more active and have shorter attention spans. If this is borne out by further studies, it may help to account for some of the different ways parents, sensitive to their babies, treat them. In addition, every baby, whether boy or girl, has strongly individual characteristics to which parents respond.

*Schedules:* "Mark broke me in easy. During the first few days he was so well organized about waking for feedings and sleeping at night that I felt as if he were scheduling me, not the other way around. I didn't have to decide whether to feed him 'on demand'—a system I didn't understand anyway. What a relief!

"But when he began to refuse food at feeding time, I didn't know what to do. Since we had done so well before, I felt this was his way of telling me something. When I tried to figure out what it was, I found that he was likely to be off schedule when he was not quite satisfied by me or was upset by something else. On one occasion he was catching my cold. On another he was just upset, as I was, after attending a noisy party where too many people handled him and played with him. Although he seemed to love it at the time, the upset showed for over twenty-four hours afterward."

I assured Mrs. Clay that, after the first two or three weeks, taking the baby out would do him no harm. He might be thrown off schedule temporarily, but he would also get acclimated to people more quickly that way. Just the same, the baby's upset demonstrates the sensitivity of an infant to outside influences, and it is best to keep him at home in the beginning, when he already has many adjustments to make.

When I spoke of schedules with Mrs. Clay, I told

her these exist for the sake of parents and
families as well as for babies. In the beginning, of
course, it is better to follow the baby's cues if
possible, because the first week at home is full of
stress for him. On the other hand some demands
a baby may make, such as wanting to be
breast-fed every two hours or needing to be
carried around all night, exceed what can
reasonably be expected of the already-tired
parents. In this case I urge parents to try to
establish a schedule that allows for their needs as
well as for those of the baby.

For instance, a mother usually cannot produce
an adequate supply of milk oftener than about
every three hours. Therefore if the baby is
fussing, she should stave him off with water or
"TLC" (tender loving care) or even with a pacifier
until her milk is ready.

If a baby cries a great deal during the night, his
parents' capacity to respond to him during the day
rapidly becomes impaired, so I often recommend
that parents push the baby to have his fussy
period in the early evening. This can be done by
waking him or playing actively with him or even
undressing him, just to get him going for a fussy
period *before* bedtime. Then it is likely that he
will sleep for the rest of the night.

Most young couples who are trying to "make it
alone" in their struggle to care for a new baby,
particularly a first one, go through much the same
kind of turmoil that Mr. and Mrs. Clay
experienced. They feel desperate and anxious,
lonely and afraid; such feelings are part of the
work that the adjustment to parenthood entails,

and they are to be expected. But while the young parents are in the midst of them, they may feel overwhelmed by their new responsibilities and seeming inadequacies in coping with them.

Then they may say, as Mrs. Clay did, "I thought I was the only one who's ever been so upset about being a new mother. Everyone tells you how great it is—I felt like an absolute failure!"

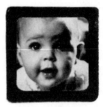

# The growing attachment

Every new mother feels some of the feelings that are described in this chapter. I realize that by saying this I may frighten a prospective mother who hasn't yet been through delivery and had experience with the postpartum blues. But the worst part of this period is the feeling of isolation and of being "queer" which young mothers experience. They feel that their depression is unique, and that they are the only ones who are inadequate to this new role. In extended family cultures, as we said before, there are ways in which the culture takes up the slack. In some parts of the world, the mother is allowed to regress to a dependent situation until she is ready to go back to work. In others, a brave front of work ethics is provided for her. She is expected to cope by returning to her work immediately. In our present situation in the United States, there is no ready-made role for the mother to step into. The week of rest in the hospital has been shortened and most young women are alone at home, with little help except their equally frightened husbands. Grandmothers are to be shunned as interferences.

In addition to the lack of support, there are increased pressures. A young woman is expected to do the perfect job of childrearing. Recent research shows that the new infant is aware of and sensitive to influences from those around him or her from the very beginning. So a new mother feels she should be entirely at the disposal of the baby. She should feel nothing but warm surges of motherliness for this new dependent creature. But then she finds it ain't so! She tries to care, but she finds herself resenting the baby, her husband, her new role!

If young mothers realize that this is a universal experience, they may not feel so queer. I always remind a new mother that worse specimens than she have made it through this period successfully.

There is a real purpose in the struggles of the recovery period. I see this period as a learning period—learning to cope with the ambivalent feelings that always accompany an important adjustment. No one ever can really give himself or herself up to another person without having misgivings and even some resentment. I equate the amount of ambivalence which young parents feel with the depth of their caring for the child. Whenever I meet a new father who is brave enough to express himself by saying, "What an unattractive baby! I don't see how I'll ever care about him!" I know he'll be the most hooked eventually. The harder they come, the harder they fall is indeed applicable.

The recovery period takes many weeks. I am convinced that for you parents to form a real attachment, you should expect it to take at least three months. When the infant can respond to you at four to six weeks, then you begin to feel it's worth it. Not many people can feel totally positive before six weeks. Fathers tell me that it takes them eight weeks or more to feel really close to their new babies, and I certainly felt that lag with mine. I was surprised and rather anxious that I didn't immediately feel overwhelmed with affection for our babies. But I didn't, and the harder I tried, the less I felt. I am sure it takes time, and all of the physical and mental struggles that go on for the first two or three months, before it comes easily. I never like to see new parents separated from their child—by day care, by nannies, by any kind of substitute caretaker— before this cycle is complete. Otherwise, they will never really feel the kind of attachment to the baby that begins when he or she looks up at you to smile and gurgle, as if you were the only important person in the world.

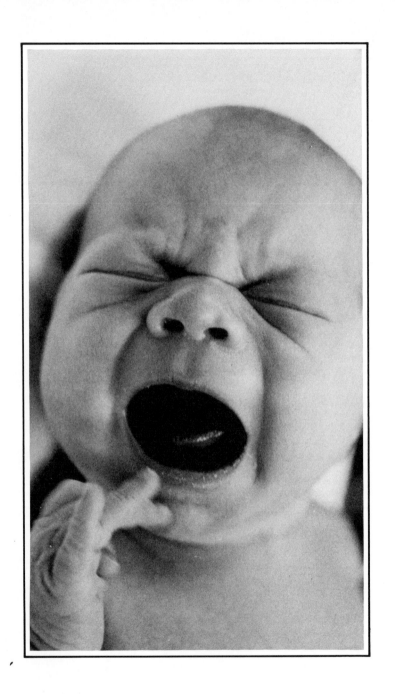

# Chapter 4

# "Colic"

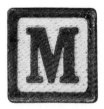y last impression of Mrs. Crane as she was about to leave the hospital with her second baby, a little girl named Lucy, was that of a relaxed, gay young woman. During my final visit to her at the lying-in hospital, she had spent most of the time discussing her older boy, Tom, and how she would handle his reaction to the new baby. She seemed confident about caring for Lucy, and I reminded her only briefly of some of the problems that might come up. We skipped lightly over my usual "crying advice."

Mrs. Crane called me once soon after she was settled in at home, with questions about a feeding schedule. She was breast-feeding Lucy and finding it a bit difficult to meet the baby's increasing demands. She also was concerned that Lucy was choking down air with her feedings. Because she

felt this would be alleviated by bubbling Lucy
more often, she had chopped the feeding periods
into little bits, feeding her a few minutes at a
time and then bubbling her. Each feeding lasted a
period of two hours. Mrs. Crane reminded me that
Tom had eaten and slept with reliable regularity
throughout his newborn period, so she was even
more upset by Lucy's crankiness.

I remembered that Mrs. Crane had nursed Tom
efficiently and pleasurably for nine months, and I
was pretty sure she had enough milk for Lucy. So
we talked about the difficulties that arise when a
vigorous baby sucks so hard at the breast that she
gulps down air with each suck. I gave her the
usual advice for such a problem: She should try to
express some of the first gushes of her milk to
avoid Lucy's having to choke it down. I also
suggested that after the feeding she prop up Lucy
at a forty-five-degree angle for a short while
before she was bubbled. This would allow gravity
to help push the air to the top of her stomach.

Because I felt that Mrs. Crane would wear
herself out if she tried to feed the baby as often as
every two hours, that she could even lose her milk
with fatigue, I urged her to try to press Lucy to
wait before each feeding. A fifteen-minute period
of fussing before a feed might serve to wake up
Lucy and thus make her suck longer when she
did get to the breast. Mrs. Crane seemed satisfied
with my suggestions and a bit relieved that I felt
nothing was wrong with her milk. She added that
Tom was "no problem" at all, as if to reassure me
that she wasn't too upset.

The next call was on the day of Lucy's
three-week birthday. Mrs. Crane was distraught,
weeping, and I could barely gather the details of
the problem. Apparently she had not slept for
thirty-six hours; Lucy had been crying off and on
most of that time, looking around for short
periods when she wasn't crying. Whenever Lucy
slept, and even when she was awake, she would
startle and then begin to cry with loud, piercing
wails.

Mrs. Crane described how the three adults in
the household—her husband, her mother, and
herself—would rush to the baby and frantically
institute a long series of efforts to quiet her down.
Lucy would refuse a pacifier. Carrying her and
rocking her quieted her briefly, but she started
again if the motion stopped. Swaddling her made
her angrier. She spat out sugar water and had
begun to refuse any bottle offered her. If she were
put to breast, she sucked briefly, choked, and
turned away after a few minutes to wail again. As
the tension in the family built up, Lucy's crying
became more frequent and more persistent. When
she did sleep it was only in short bursts, and then
Tom had been up and making demands.

Mrs. Crane's mother and her husband had
blamed her milk for Lucy's "colic" and had urged
her to wean her to some "decent food" so that the
child would settle down. Mrs. Crane was ready to
give up nursing, but she felt that this would not
be the answer to Lucy's crying. She thought that
Lucy was a baby she could not understand. In
fact, she was so desperate that she feared she

might hurt Lucy in anger if she didn't find a
solution to the crying.

Mrs. Crane sounded depleted, frantic. Although
she asked for my advice, when I made suggestions
she barely listened. Her mother came to the
phone to ask me for sedative medication for the
baby. I suggested that that would not be a
solution, but my words were falling on deaf ears.

I decided to pay the Cranes a visit at home, for I
was familiar with the "colic syndrome" and knew
that when family tensions had reached these
dimensions, the most effective way to deal with
them was for all of us—all three generations and
myself—to sort it out together.

When I arrived I found the house disorganized,
Mrs. Crane bedraggled, her mother frantically
hovering, Tom crying, and the new baby wailing
while the exhausted father walked her to and fro.
I sat down in a rocking chair to hold the baby,
and as I rocked she quieted in my arms and
looked up at me. Babies are sensitive to tension in
the air and often are soothed easily by an
objective newcomer who is not so keyed up as
they. I used this dramatic period of peace to talk
to the family.

After examining Lucy I could assure them that
she was neither ill nor hungry. Feeling the
tension in her body as I held her, feeling her
startle from time to time as I rocked her, I knew
that she was one of those infants who seem to use
crying as a method of letting off steam, of exercise
and activity, of reaching out to the environment
in much the same way a quieter baby might look

around or suck placidly on his or her fists. I could predict that Lucy, like all babies, would cry a total of at least three hours a day over the next nine weeks in spite of all attempts to quiet her. I also could assure the parents that their own anxiety and frustration when they weren't able to quiet her would be transmitted to her, fueling her crying, making her "colicky."

From a necessary three hours of crying, colicky babies begin to build up to eight or twelve hours a day. As they cry, their entire body, including the intestinal tract, becomes tense and overactive. They gulp down air as they cry. Their stomach is sensitive to it and it creates pain, so they cry harder. As they pass the gas on through the rectum, the pain persists, and so does the crying. Colic is usually blamed on the infant's gastrointestinal tract. I am convinced, however, that the physiological involvement is secondary to the buildup of tension in the whole body.

To relieve the vicious circle that was developing in Lucy, I urged the family members to try to relax and get more sleep. I encouraged Mrs. Crane to keep on with her breast feeding but to avoid strong foods, which might possibly upset Lucy (although I'm convinced few foods do upset a colicky baby). I urged her to try to get more rest between feedings and thus allow her breasts to recover after each one in order to build up her milk supply. I repeated the earlier advice I had given about reducing the ingestion of air at feeding times and propping up Lucy to look around before she was bubbled. And then I

begged all three adults to stop their frantic
fussing over her.

I assured them it was not as hard on her to cry
for periods of fifteen to twenty minutes at a time
before being picked up as it was to be jostled and
held with no message coming across but one of
frantic tension. I assured them that if she cried
for short bursts, was given sugar water, and
bubbled periodically, the water would mobilize
whatever air she had cried down and sucking on
the bottle would quiet her. I asked them to set up
just such a routine when she was colicky—twenty
minutes of crying, ten minutes of sucking and
comforting, twenty minutes more of crying, and so
on. They were to keep a log of the day and call
me each afternoon to report on the crying.

Within five days Lucy's crying was organized
into two predictable periods: one hour in the early
morning and two more at suppertime. Although
she had a few periods of ten-minute-long wails at
other times, she was over them before the parents
could feed the sugar water. We had cured Lucy's
colic *before* she was three months old.

I am pretty convinced that much of the "colic"
that new babies have is based on the interaction
between a tense, hyperactive baby and a pair of
frustrated, exhausted parents. However, there
certainly are many reasons why new babies cry
that can be tragically missed if one labels all
crying as colic. I do not believe that a baby should
be left to "cry it out" until the parents have made
every possible attempt to find the reasons and to
quiet him or her. But when parents find that their

remedies are adding to the baby's problems, it is time to let the baby help find his or her own solution!

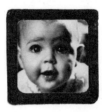

# The normal crying period

When I first started practicing pediatrics, about half of my morning phone calls were concerned with babies' crying. Frantic young mothers called me day after day for a magical solution to their problem, and I kept offering them one solution after another. I too was caught up with their conviction that, "if only we do the right thing," the baby would be satisfied, and would quiet down. I tried all of the solutions offered in the textbooks, in the mothers' magazines, in the pharmacy manuals. We swaddled, we used pacifiers, we used rocking chairs, we used sedatives. Each attempt seemed to work at first, but very quickly began to fail. And the infants seemed to go on crying relentlessly day after day. When mothers became worn out and frantic themselves, the babies cried more and more.

As a last resort, I began to ask some of these parents to keep me daily charts of how much crying their infants had really done, what time of day, what efforts they'd made to quiet the baby, and with what outcome. I was able to learn several important things from these charts. The

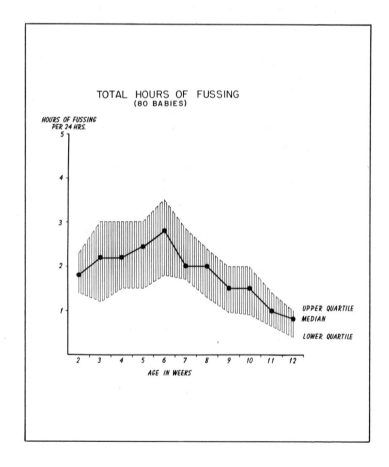

first was that, although it seemed to the parents
that the baby was crying all day and all night, the
truth was that the total crying did not amount to
more than two hours a day. The second important
observation was that the more frantic maneuvers
a mother used to try to quiet him, the more the
baby cried. The third was that if the parents
could allow for a certain amount of crying and
intersperse their own quiet, calm attempts to
soothe the infant periodically, the crying settled
down to the expectable two hours a day. This
period of crying began to decrease over time and
by ten weeks was just about gone. By twelve
weeks, at the very same period of the day, the
infant was sociable, gay, and vocalizing. It almost
appeared that this crying period was the
precursor of a sociable period. It quickly became
apparent that a certain amount of fussing at the
end of each day was inevitable in most infants in
the period from three to ten weeks. The graph
shows the amount of crying that was recorded for
eighty "normal" babies.

Armed with this information, I have revised my
opinion that there is an easy solution to an
infant's crying. At certain times of the day, babies
seem to need to cry and efforts to soothe them
may be in vain. With this conviction, I have been
able to reassure most new parents that their
problems with a crying infant are not unique, nor
is there a magical way to solve them, except over
time. The end to these crying periods seems to
come when the baby can do other, more
interesting things—such as cooing, smiling,
babbling, and so on. Meanwhile in the first three

months, the crying period seems to be a channel for the baby's energies, a time to let off steam, an exercise period, and so on. I saw the same two hours of crying in a group of Mayan Indian babies whose mothers swaddled and carried them all day, slept next to them all night, and breast-fed them thirty to forty times a day on "demand." None of these maneuvers was a panacea for a baby's crying. A crying period at the end of each day seems to be almost universal for babies.

I would now urge a mother or father in charge of a newborn who has started to cry more and more first to try the things that might quiet him or her—that is, feeding, changing, cuddling, rocking, or a finger or a pacifier to suck on. But then, if none of these work, the important thing is not to get excited. This is probably a normal crying period for the baby, and it may be just as inevitable a part of the day as feedings and sleep. When parents can accept this, they do not add their tension to the baby's, and increase the need for crying.

There are a certain number of infants who are more sensitive to outside stimuli than the average. They respond with an unusual amount of crying and motor activity and become very difficult for their parents. They cry more than two hours a day, are difficult to quiet, and they overreact to everything that occurs around them. The job for parents with these babies is even greater—they *must* develop a calm routine in order to calm these babies. Otherwise, these hyperreactive babies can become fussier and fussier over the

first twelve weeks, and indeed become "colicky."
They can cry as much as twelve hours a day.
They will survive but their parents won't.
Follow-up studies on some of these overreactive
infants show that they often grow up to be
extremely bright, alert children—if their parents
can learn techniques for handling them in this
early period.

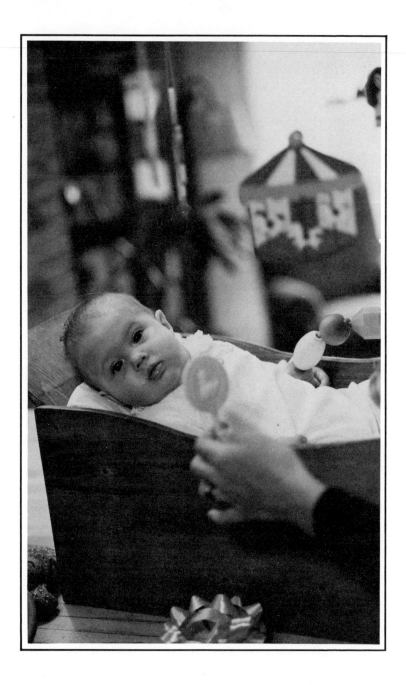

## Chapter 5

# Are there too many sights and sounds in your baby's world?

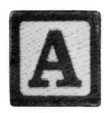newborn baby lies in his, or her, crib in the hospital nursery. Noise surrounds him as nurses talk and infants cry. But our baby isn't disturbed. He continues as he was, resting peacefully in his crib, breathing slowly and steadily—eyes open, looking around, or eyes shut, asleep. Try clapping your hands near him. He may startle briefly or he may not respond even that much—he may just shut it all out.

But if you shake a soft rattle near his ear or speak softly to him, his face will become alert, his regular breathing will change to irregular and he will gradually turn his head in the direction of the "attractive" noise. Moreover, if a man speaks on one side and a higher-pitched female voice competes on the other, the baby will turn toward the female voice.

If you flash a bright-yellow light into the baby's

closed eyes, he will blink and then shut it out completely. But if you use a soft-red light, he will gradually rouse from sleep and begin to look for the source. Then if you slowly—at his speed—move the light, he will turn his head to follow it from side to side, and even up and down.

The ability to shut out loud noises and bright light is part of the marvelous equipment that every human being is born with. It means that from the time of birth a baby is very much aware of what goes on around him, that he can tune in or tune out on his environment, that he can respond to the stimuli around him or reject them, that he can sort out what is "appropriate" and what is not. And once he makes his choice of stimuli, certain responses are immediately set in motion.

In the examples above we saw how the baby instinctually turned toward the attractive sounds and the attractive voice. And he is capable of other kinds of behavior that are much more complex. For instance, when a mother offers her baby milk, either from her breast or from a bottle, and she strokes his cheek, the baby will "root"— that is, turn his head toward the source—until he finds the nipple. He will then shut out all interfering activity and aim his whole body toward getting the milk.

All this may seem so obvious to you that it's not particularly impressive, but you may change your mind if you take a look at the rest of the baby's behavior. He stops sucking from time to time to look up at his mother and around the room. During these brief pauses the mother speaks to her baby, strokes or caresses him and rocks him gently. But instead of urging him back to suck, the mother's gestures seem to produce longer pauses as the baby drinks in these other kinds of stimulation from her.

In this way the baby builds up a whole Gestalt, or combination of cues, which he associates with being fed, with being mothered in a particular way. And so powerful do these cues become that by the time the baby is four weeks old, he may be unwilling to eat properly without them.

One young father told me that he was feeding his month-old baby a bottle when the baby heard his mother's voice. The baby stopped sucking and refused to return to the bottle. This demonstrated to me—and to the father—the power of the association that important cues can build up. Fortunately, however, the baby does not limit his powers of association to the feeding experience only. He develops an increasing awareness of the importance of other cues and other situations.

Although this father was a bit disconcerted by his baby's demand for the special nursing situation his wife had provided, he was proudly aware of the strength it represented. And this was easy to demonstrate in other ways. Once in my office, when the father held the baby and talked to him, the baby's face lighted up in a series of smiles, as if he were saying, "I'm ready to play." But when his mother held him and tried to talk to him, he began to look serious and to root, as if he expected to be fed.

The human infant is surely endowed with the ability to take in, to store, and to learn important

things from his environment as soon as he is
born. And it is essential that the environment give
the infant the chance to do just that.

There are three forces that propel an infant
from one stage of development to the next: an
instinctual drive to survive, no matter how
complex the world may seem; a drive toward
mastery of himself and his world, which can best
be seen in the excitement he expresses as he
makes each developmental step: and finally the
need to fit into, to identify with, and to become
part of his environment.

The first two drives—for survival and for
mastery—come from within the infant. The third
force comes from the environment. The
stimulation of sights and sounds and especially of
the people around the baby shape his or her inner
drives and responses. If the environment is sterile
or nonresponsive, the other drives will either
come to a standstill or wither away.

Just as a baby needs proper nutrients for
physiological growth, he or she depends on
stimulation for emotional and intellectual growth.
Lack of stimulation is, then, a devastating kind of
experience, because it can interfere with
development. And we have only to look at what
happens to infants living in institutions to see
this.

Institutionalized children may be fed, changed,
and talked to on schedule, but when their
demands for attention are not met at their own
tempo, their responses become less frequent and
their demands less forceful. Their cries become
weaker, their smiles fade, and they turn inward.

They begin to roll their heads, play weakly with their hands or hair or clothes, and stare at the walls with an empty look. Their responses to their caretaker consist of an apathetic curiosity or anxiety, which they demonstrate by turning toward the wall or hiding behind their hands. As their needs and demands are not met when they express them, their expectations for a response begin to dwindle. Thus the basis for failure is set up; the vicious circle becomes established.

Without the feedback of demand-response from their environment, these babies will not generate the energy to develop properly. They can appear to be mentally defective, or autistic, by the age of six months—and condemned to a hopeless institutionalization for life.

Can this happen in a "normal" environment? Probably not—because I am convinced that a great deal that a sensitive mother does, which is, as far as she is concerned, just part of being a mother, contributes immeasurably to developing her child's responsiveness. But even the most sensitive mothers may want some guidance. And by knowing more about the mechanisms your baby uses to select what he or she can use and shut out what he or she cannot use, perhaps you can create an even more stimulating environment.

But first let me warn you about two practical dangers, something that even experts can overlook —overstimulation and inappropriate stimulation.

A very good example of what I mean by overstimulation comes from an eminent researcher in infancy who set up an experiment with eight-week-old babies. He put into their cribs special pillows, so constructed that when the babies turned their heads in a certain direction, mobiles suspended directly overhead would move. Within a few weeks the infants realized that the movement of the mobile depended on their activity; they cooed with pleasure and were willing to lie in bed for long periods, making the mobile turn.

The speed with which the infants realized their role in the mobile's movement, as well as the joy they took in such realization, delighted everyone. That is, until it was seen that not only were the infants willing to produce this activity for long periods, but many of them were hooked on it— they ate and slept better when they were attached to the apparatus.

Now we come to my second concern—the necessity that stimulation be appropriate for each particular baby. My worst dream about this was realized at a demonstration at the American Academy of Pediatrics, where doctors were shown all the new toys that can be used to provide a "stimulating environment" for infants. One crib, specially set up, was a nightmare of dangling, projecting, moving, musical toys—toys that would attack a poor infant from every side, through all the senses. I wanted to place an infant in the midst of all this in order to show how powerful are the defense mechanisms of the human organism. I know what the baby would have done —gone to sleep!

But this demonstration was urged as an example of how mothers could improve on their

babies' environment—and the advertising that
accompanied these toys implied that unless a
mother provided such stimuli, she was neglecting
opportunities for her infant. In other words, she
was unknowingly being a "bad" mother.

I saw the mobile as a potentially harmful
weapon that at worst might lead infants to turn
away from their world and at best might teach
them to handle the overpowering stimulation of
an assaultive technological society. I worried most
about the effect this kind of brainwashing has on
mothers and fathers, for the implication was that
experts have answers parents must follow blindly
if they are to provide an optimal climate for their
infant's development. I don't buy that, for I
believe that most parents are in a better position
to provide the environment that is suited to their
baby and his or her needs.

I admit that sometimes I have seen mothers
who, in their eagerness to provoke a reaction or
simply to gain attention from their baby, failed to
realize that the stimulation they were offering
*was* excessive or inappropriate. I've seen this
happen for a period of months—the mother
overstimulating, the baby withdrawing—without
the mother's realizing it, until I finally stepped in
to interpret the baby's behavior.

I have two major worries when this kind of
thing goes on too long, and it is these that help
me overcome my reluctance to interfere in a
relationship. First, I fear the baby will eventually
build up some kind of strategy for dealing with
Mother or some kind of expectancy regarding her

that makes him or her eventually think, Oh, *her!*
She wants me to perform again! and almost
automatically withdraw as soon as he or she sees
her coming. Second, I worry that the mother may
quite suddenly take to heart her failure to reach
her baby and, feeling futile or rejected, summarily
switch from providing too much or too
inappropriate stimulation to providing too little.
In this case the baby may lose out on intellectual
as well as emotional aspects of development.

But how can a mother fail to realize that the
stimulation she is offering her infant is excessive
or inappropriate? I think all mothers can tell
when they have made a hit, for the baby's
alerting eyes or smile or the turning of the head
toward her tells her that. Similarly there are very
few mothers who are incapable of getting the
opposite message if a baby cries or actively tries
to squirm away. Some babies, however, have ways
of withdrawing that are more subtle—and some
mothers are less ready as interpreters.

Let me tell you in detail about two of my
favorite patients—I think you'll see at once why
this baby and his mother are that. I'm thinking of
a charming and high-geared young woman who
talks, thinks, and reads as quickly as she moves,
and whose very stacatto beat was the charisma
that attracted her solid, thoughtful, and careful,
slow-moving husband. They had a baby, Michael,
and since Michael was like her husband, the
mother naturally treated him to the same urgent
and high-speed maneuvers.

In his earliest months I used to watch Michael
in his infant seat on my desk. He sat looking

around, stolid and quietly satisfied. I thought that
he was particularly alert to low-geared sounds
and voices. I watched him brighten and turn to
soft, slow voices and show real pleasure when I
turned on a quiet music box. But in those days his
mother wanted him to *do* something—*quick!*
Moreover, I was aware that she not only wanted
him to react or give some kind of performance,
such as grasping an object, but also would have
liked him to accomplish certain motor feats
earlier than most babies.

I watched the mother "play" with him. She
fluttered about him and gaily, rapidly, and
persistently poked, patted, and shook him and
darted back and forth in front of him with
birdlike movements. I watched Michael in his
own way, over a period of minutes and then of
weeks, withdraw from her high-pressure tactics.
His eyes would become heavy-lidded, his face
dull, and his whole body sink heavily into the
infant seat as she continued to nuzzle and
impatiently urge him. She interpreted this
tuning-out reaction to her ministrations
alternately as stupidity or sleepiness.

It soon became clear, however, that there was
no question of stupidity, for Michael, so alert to
sounds and voices, first cooed, then vocalized
happily in little conversations with his father,
who usually would wait patiently for an interested
response to his last maneuver before attempting
the next. And I saw how well his gentle, shy,
patient manner paid off.

Michael's mother was upset by her own failure
and her husband's success, so we discussed the

difference in their approach. I pointed out to her
that there *is* a kind of sleepiness that even in
newborns is a reaction to excessive stimulation. I
told her of my experiences with infants who
suddenly fall into a deep sleep during an
examination or after an inoculation.

It was as though, rather than physically getting
away from obnoxious or excessive stimulation, the
infants were seeing to it that the stimulation had
less power over them. They were increasing the
inner distance between them and it. I told her I
thought her little boy's sleepy apathy might be
somehow related to that kind of entirely healthy,
but defensive, response. She listened.

Of course I told her that only her own alertness
to her baby's individuality could tell her which
particular kinds as well as quantities of
stimulation were especially for him; that of course
there are no recipes. Finally I told her that now
that she realized she had a quiet, nonmotoric baby
on her hands, one who liked to be talked to, she
might look for other cues in his behavior—
perhaps the fact that he was more responsive
before dinner than after. She was able to take this
advice to heart and use it.

At the next visit they were a unit! The mother
was quieter, more sensitive to Michael and his
reactions, and Michael was more actively
responsive to her as she talked to him. He whirled
his arms, arched forward toward her, gurgled
with delight, and cooed back to her. In a month
they both had changed, and they were off to an
increasingly exciting relationship!

Infants are usually slower to act and slower to react than older children, and clearly are slower than adults. I've often thought that must be why we talk to them and handle them as we do. Baby talk is one example. Certainly we say, "Good morning, Jeffrey; how are you?" quite differently to our babies from the way we do to our peers. Perhaps we are sensitively adjusting our input to the ability of babies to take it in. We pitch our voices to appeal to their preference for higher-pitched sounds and to signal that now we are talking to them. We slow down as we speak so that we can fit into their slower rhythms.

When a mother fails to slow down for her baby, she disturbs him by presenting information too quickly for him to absorb it. On those occasions, when he does manage to take it in, a mother may also fail to give him time to respond; so even if the baby does finally give some indication that her behavior has been interesting, pleasant, and appropriate, she may well have gone on impatiently to something else.

I've seen mothers trying to get a smile out of a young baby, obviously expecting that if he or she had a mind to, the baby could smile as easily and quickly as her adult friends. This isn't true, and I've often had the experience of watching an impatient mother turn away just as her baby *is* smiling—now into thin air.

Another thing that has fascinated me for some time is the periodicity of a child's attention. In my work with detailed film analysis at Harvard's Center for Cognitive Research, I have found that during an interval as short as a minute an infant whose gaze had seemed to the naked eye to have been fastened steadily on the mother (whose instructions were to interact with the infant) had actually averted it an average of six times a minute. In other words, there were six cycles of attending and withdrawing in one minute of intense interaction. It was as though the infant needed brief periods of respite.

Furthermore I found that the more sensitive mothers, usually without realizing it, had leaned back, ceased talking, or averted their own gaze during those brief intervals, waiting for their children's own cue that they were ready to communicate with them again. A less sensitive mother might have kept up a steady barrage of input during this period, or even intensified her behavior in response to the baby's withdrawal.

The educator John Holt has noted this kind of cycling activity on a much grander scale and in older children. He watched two different parents trying to teach their toddlers to swim. One tried steadily, overriding the child's need to stop at brief intervals and perhaps just survey the situation with the aid of a steadying hand. The scene ended in distress. The second parent allowed the child, at his own timing, to put his head in the water and bravely make his little arm strokes and then turn to cling to his father for reassurance. Perhaps he needed not only to withdraw briefly from his efforts, but also to be assured again of his father's presence.

A mother, of course, functions as a secure base for her infant's little explorations into the world.

Without her presence a baby takes far less interest in exploration. With it he or she may repeatedly sally forth to learn about toys, strange persons, and furniture—but after a few brief minutes seems to need assurance of her presence, will return repeatedly to her side or call to her before once more moving forth to learn about the world. When a relationship is going well, there is a lovely, easy, rhythmic quality to the baby's movements away from and back to the mother. And the mother's accessibility seems to contribute tremendously to the courage to learn.

By repeatedly noticing and responding to her baby's wants, needs, and expectations, a mother gives the "pleasure of being the cause"—of learning how to act in order to produce the results he or she wants, of learning about things that are the results of his or her own actions. Here is real learning! It takes place with great rapidity, it is accompanied by real joy, and for many months of life it is dependent largely upon the mother. Since inanimate objects cannot respond to a baby's unspoken cues, since they do not whirl, sing, or come to the baby's bidding on their own, the mother must act as intermediary.

She must stand between her baby and his world, interpreting, patient and sensitive. This is true mothering.

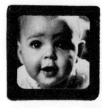 # Overstimulation

Today, mothers of even the tiniest infants seem overly concerned about how much "teaching" they should be doing. They have heard that one must be aware of the stages of development through which each infant proceeds, and that a parent should be offering stimulation appropriate to that stage. Implied in this presently accepted notion is the belief that if you miss an opportunity, your baby may not be able to compete with his or her neighbors and peers. One commonly stated warning is that if babies don't crawl before they walk, they may be handicapped later on, so you must "teach" them to crawl. Mothers are also urged to teach their children to read at even earlier ages. "Sesame Street" teaches two and a half-year-olds their letters. Many parents today are urging two- and three-year-olds on to reading words. I have had several four-year-old children in my practice who could indeed read long sentences, and could type out words on a typewriter, spelling them correctly as they did so. The parents of such children are proud, for a lot of pressure from them has gone into the child's achievement. And the neighbors of these children all feel "put down," as if they had neglected their own children by not pushing them into such early achievement. "Contingent reinforcement" is a phrase that is bandied about rather freely in the psychological world today. A mother who greets each of her child's productions with an immediate, encouraging response is reinforcing his or her behavior and is doing it contingently— soon after the child's behavior. As a result, the child is led to know that this particular behavior is prized. Contingent reinforcement presses a child on to repeat the behavior again—and again. In this way, children learn rapidly—often even before they are ready—to perform more and more complex tasks. A parent who "leads" a baby on in this way is considered a good middle-class parent by psychologists. By the same token, one who does not isn't doing her best for the infant. Mothers and fathers are immersed in the guilty feeling that if they don't press their infants onward, they will lag behind in the race for first grade or nursery school. No one in the middle-class population in which I practice can stand to take a chance on the child's getting behind. Their own lives are full of competition, and striving hard is part of their way of life. So, this eager, early teaching and prodding can become a primary mode of interaction between parents and their children.

What is lost in this kind of approach to parenting? The most serious danger to me is that children may not be allowed to pace themselves or to find their own way to a new skill. And since they learn each task under pressure, there is no real sense of mastery or self-fulfillment on which to pride themselves. Perhaps the praise they gather makes up for not having the rewarding feeling of having achieved a task for themselves, but I doubt it. One need only think of the utter delight on a baby's face as he or she takes a first step. If that delight is subtracted from each new step in development, I don't believe that parental praise can really match it.

In addition, an environment full of pressure to learn is likely to become a strained, joyless one. Too many of us have ourselves under pressure and will transmit it unconsciously to our children. To add conscious pressure to learn each task really does seem pretty unnecessary. The world in which children in our culture will grow up is a high-pressured one, and the pressures on them will be enormous as soon as they are in school. Does it seem reasonable to start this pressure in the first year? Not to me. A few parents justify their early pressure by saying that children will have to learn how to deal with it later, so they might as well begin early.

My main concern about the current pressure on small children to learn is that we really don't know which ingredients of a child's development should be uppermost at these ages. It would seem to me that a small child's major task must be to learn to live with himself or herself and with those around. In the second and third years, children must learn how to get along with their peers. If the pressure to learn were indeed aimed at these tasks, I could feel they were more appropriate to children's development. Children left to their own devices learn via play—both alone and with others near their own age. For those parents who feel they must listen to the cognitively directed experts, I would urge that they balance their early teaching with a large dose of affectionate encouragement for the child's own joy in learning by himself or herself.

The preceding article was designed to alert parents to the signals that small children can give when they have had enough! I hope it will help to add balance to their world, and to give the children of our generation more time for joy and for peace of mind than we have allowed ourselves.

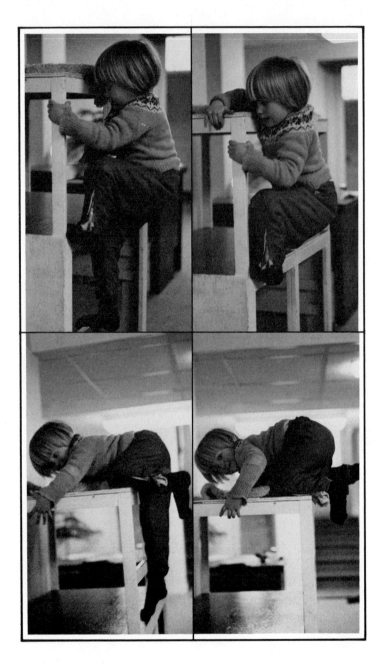

*Chapter 6*

# The children
# who can't sit still

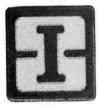n the newborn nursery in a large
maternity hospital, a nurse called
my attention to one of the babies
she'd been feeding. "I think you'd
better warn the mother," the nurse
said, "that she will have a rough
time settling this boy down."

When a busy nurse is struck by the behavior of
one of the many babies she is in charge of, I have
learned to listen carefully to her observations. Not
only do they accurately assess unusual behavior
in the infant, but also they often are important
predictions of how he or she will act later on.
When the nurse warned me that this baby was
"hard to quiet," I was sure he would be
exceptionally so when he was taken home.

With the nurse's comments in mind, I watched
the child myself for a period, and my observations
were as follows:

When he slept, he slept so lightly that almost any noise or movement awakened him.

When he awakened, he awakened suddenly with a cry and a startle that built up rapidly to screaming and thrashing.

When he was crying, very little would calm him down. In fact, every attempt to quiet him seemed to make him cry harder.

When he was awake but not crying, any slight noise or jolt startled him; and the vicious circle of crying, startling, and then crying because of his startles was set up.

When he thrashed, his legs and arms cycled wildly and without real purpose. He often fought until he was exhausted and then fell suddenly into his light sleep.

When his attention was caught by a bright toy or soft music, he couldn't look or listen for more than a moment before he started to cry.

Now, these kinds of behavior might describe any new baby from time to time, for all infants have periods of crying in which nothing seems to work to quiet them. In the first two months at home, especially, there usually are three or four hours of determined fussing each day that mothers and fathers can't control or can only alleviate for rather brief periods. Many newborns start this fussing in the hospital. But if the parents can "teach" these babies how to develop ways of dealing with their overreactions, most of them gradually begin to calm down. By the end of the third month they have "learned" ways of coping with the environment and themselves and are no longer difficult.

It is with the parents of those few babies who *don't* settle down as they mature, who seem to be more driven rather than less as they turn the three-month corner, that I am most concerned here, for the parents of these children need extra help. Hyperactive infants are hard to live with. They can develop into intense, hyperactive children who cannot calm themselves down, who cannot concentrate for long on any one thing, who overreact to every intervention from the outside as if it were a challenge to more violent activity, and whose excessive demands produce angry, guilty reactions in their young parents. I am hoping this article will let these parents see that their baby's difficult behavior is not all their fault and that there are ways of coping with it that may help them and the baby over the long haul. At the very least they may see that they are not all alone in their despair.

A young mother brought her four-month-old infant, Dan, into my office. She was close to tears. She had been trying desperately to breast-feed him, but she was so exhausted and distraught that her milk was almost gone. She described her life at home during the past four months: Her husband blamed her for being too tense; her mother kept saying that the baby must be hungry; her two-year-old son, Tom, was sad and neglected, clinging to her skirts all day long as she busied herself with the new baby.

"Dan wakes up screaming every three hours, day and night," she said. "He never lies in bed watching his mobile or his hands. When he sees

me, he screams even louder. If I pick him up, he
turns to cry in my ear. When I put him to my
breast, he turns away from it, and I have to force
him to take the nipple. When he finally starts
sucking, any little noise from Tom startles him,
and he drops the nipple to cry. If I try to feed him
solids, he chokes. If I give him a bottle, he
splutters, gulps, and then spits up. I feel like a
hopeless failure.

"Tom was never like this. He was active and
cried some every day, but I could understand him.
This baby can't enjoy anything. When I finally get
him quiet after a feeding, by swaddling him so he
won't be so jumpy, he may finally start to watch
or listen to something. All of a sudden he is
startled, and he's off into his loud, impenetrable
crying. I get so desperate that I want to smother
him or put him so far away I can't hear him. I'm
afraid I might drop him or hurt him. I can't stand
this baby!"

As she told me her story Dan began to scream
in her arms. I thought to myself, He is surely
sensitive to her being upset, and I offered to take
him from her. In my arms he became rigid,
stiffening like an arched board. When I looked
into his face, he screamed, shut his eyes, and
turned away. He wailed solidly as I tried to cradle,
to cuddle, to rock, and to soothe him. When I
crooned to him, he shut me out with louder wails.
It took a great deal of effort just to keep him from
dropping out of my arms. Indeed, he was giving
me a real demonstration of how hard it would be
to try to love him. I realized in these few minutes
why Dan's mother was so desperate.

During pregnancy every mother has a picture of herself in harmony with her new baby. The baby is some sort of idealized version of her friends' children and the models she sees in magazines. Of course, no real baby ever fits a mother's preconceptions, but most babies do respond in subtle, satisfying ways to the efforts of even a new mother. When you hold him, he cuddles into the crook of your arm. When you sing to him, his face softens and alerts and he turns to look up at you. During a feeding he gradually relaxes and smooths down into a cycle of sucking and contented looking around.

Such periods create a bond of attachment between you and your baby that help you through the trying periods. When there never are such harmonious times to build upon, when you get so little feedback from your baby, you must *force* yourself to like him. But the efforts you make to reach him all seem to turn him away.

He makes you feel inadequate, but as you begin to be angry with yourself and with him for your helplessness, you realize he is only a baby and doesn't deserve the hostile feelings he is generating in you. The only thing you are left with then is a mixture of desperation and guilt.

I was tempted to try to reassure this young mother, to tell her to have patience and that "Dan would outgrow it." But I also knew that wasn't enough. And if I didn't do more to help, I was contributing in my own way to the vicious circle that was beginning to close in on her and her family. How could I protect them from disintegrating in the face of such a demanding child?

This mother needed an understanding of her baby as a person who was separate from her; she needed to know what he was likely to do when he overreacted to her handling. Most important, she needed to know that his hyperactivity was not her fault, that it was a part of his own makeup. She needed to know that she could learn ways to handle him that eventually would calm him down and lead to his learning how to handle his own tension and high-geared reactions. It was likely to be a long and wearing road ahead for her, for her husband, and for their other child.

I thought of other patients I'd known who were like Dan. There was one-year-old Matthew, constantly on the go. He'd charge all over the house, disregarding everything in his path. His mother said that he leaned forward, set his course, and propelled one leg after another as if he were on a downhill course to his goal. He fell over everything that got in his way, hitting his head with loud whacks that brought everyone running. Nothing seemed to bother him except the frustration of being blocked.

When he was put in a high chair to be fed, he blew up with angry cries. When he was given a spoon or a cup, he hurled them away. He broke all his toys in rapid succession. His investigations carried him upstairs to tumble backward down them, into closets to find mothballs to eat, into the laundry cupboard to drink detergent—constantly moving from one trap to another. His mother and father spent most of their day keeping after him.

When they brought him in for a checkup, they were unable to take their eyes off him. Every

move he made toward an object in my office
brought them up to a rigid, watching position.
They were after him at every move, and our
discussions about him were peppered with their
commands to him—which he ignored.

More ominously, they had been short and
abrupt with each other. The anger and the tension
Matthew was creating in them they now aimed at
each other. As a result, they themselves were
making the home environment tenser and more
stressful. And of course Matthew responded to this
by being even more active and irritable, which
only fueled the already deterioriating situation.

I remembered another session recently with
John, who is now eight. His parents have been
through years of concern and are exhausted. John
too is depressed about himself, although he can
barely express it. He tries so hard—too hard—to
please, with an ingratiating smile, correct
manners, and a plea on his face for you to like
him. His appeal turns into a transient
obsequiousness as he begins to shuffle his feet, to
finger his clothes, to look off into the distance in
an effort to control his energy to listen to you.
Soon he is away, darting from one part of the
room to another, unable to stand or sit still any
longer.

He looks unhappy when his face is not in jerky
motion like the rest of his body. He has a
hangdog, beaten look, as if he felt defeated by his
own inadequacies. He says about himself: "None
of the kids can stand me because I'm so clumsy. I
can't catch a ball. I can't even build a tower of
blocks. I can't learn how to add. All I can do is be

silly to make them laugh. But they don't laugh at me—they just tease."

His parents are despairing because he has been unable to make any academic progress in school. They have moved him from one school to another to try to find an atmosphere where he can learn. In the big public school he attended, he met with everyone's disapproval, disrupting classes by his inability to sit still and his constantly distracting behavior. The teachers say he's "impossible and never will learn."

But the fact is that he's not stupid. Psychological tests indicated that he functions well above average, except in tasks that require organized thinking and motor performance. In other words, he demonstrated islands of really superior intelligence that showed through a pretty disorganized performance.

John's parents spend their time watching him fearfully. They alternate between giving him constant directions and sighing in anguish as they try to control their desperation.

I wonder how to help Dan's parents *before* they reach such an impasse. Are there things they can do to cut down on the tension around him? Can they see him as a normal but active child? Is he really normal, or does he suffer some form of mild brain damage that shows up in him as this mixture of activity and sensitivity?

Most children are hyperactive for a combination of reasons that may not be easy to diagnose. Although there does seem to be some relationship between mild brain damage and the disorganized, overreactive responses that characterize hyperactivity, a disorder of the central nervous system is thought to exist in only 8 to 10 percent of the children who are labeled "hyperactive." For the great majority of these children there is no organic impairment; but there may be a kind of behavioral disorganization and immaturity, with the result that hyperactivity and hypersensitivity are the ways these youngsters use to cope with underlying anxiety and distress.

For the 10 percent who have brain damage, amphetamine drugs seem to be effective. With the use of such drugs all the symptoms—the high energy level; the clumsy, inefficient motor activity; the distractible, hopelessly inefficient learning patterns—improve rapidly and dramatically. As these children become adolescents, particularly if they have had a chance to "learn" how to cope with their problems of disorganization, they outgrow the need for stimulant drugs without becoming addicted to or dependent on them, and the chances are good that they will mature into normal, successful adults.

Minor brain damage, I must emphasize, affects only the minority 10 percent. It can be detected only after a careful examination, usually by a specialist in the field of hyperactivity, and even then the diagnosis often is not clear until after the drug treatment works. So for the parents of most hyperactive children, drug treatment is not the answer.

This larger group of children frequently can benefit from psychotherapy. John, for example, could probably profit from this kind of help. His parents too can certainly use professional attention for their side of the interaction. Special tutoring or a learning situation that can be geared to him may redirect the energy he expresses in overreactions and distractibility into very effective learning patterns. And then a sensitive approach to helping him with his peers may give him an opportunity to learn how to cope with other children and how to handle himself in social situations.

Still, I do not think this kind of program is necessary in all cases. I would first urge a preventive approach that may help the parents of children like Dan to cope with their problems and thus avoid the difficulties that have already piled up for John and Matthew.

First of all, Dan's parents must realize that his combination of sensitivity and overreactivity is part of his temperament—it is not their fault. Certainly they can't change him into another kind of baby. Hence, comparing him to other babies will be endlessly frustrating.

The best they can do will be to help him learn how to modulate some of his reactions. Instead of trying to protect him from stimulation in the environment that may indeed upset him, they must *expect* him to respond with an overreaction. Then they can help him calm himself down, soothing him as they do it—but calmly, not with tense anxiety. They can learn to offer him quiet, subdued experiences too—and encouragement when he works hard to learn to conquer his reactions.

This will be a long and demanding job for both

of them. They must see it as such, and they must support each other. For instance, Dan's mother must plan to get away from Dan in order to preserve her own equanimity and to see herself and her son more objectively. A regular sitter will help. Dan's father must feel free to play with Dan in his own way, to try out active ways of channeling some of this energy. Although he will get frustrated too, the male-to-male relationship has a different kind of tolerance in it. Fathers usually can put up with more raw aggression and more fumbling than mothers, as long as they know that putting up with it is their part in helping the child. They too need to see the boy as a challenge, not as their failure. Of course, and it goes without saying, the importance of having an understanding father is more than pure gold for a boy like Dan.

An overactive baby like Dan may benefit from soothing treatment that would not be necessary with other babies—such as swaddling the lower half of his body before he goes to sleep or is propped in his infant chair. I would also offer him a toy to use as a "lovey" for sleep periods. He may be quieted by extra sucking, and I wouldn't hesitate to give him a pacifier, *if* he will accept it and if it has a calming effect on him. Moreover, he would profit from extra periods of being rocked and sung to at times when he is trying to quiet himself down.

I feel all these crutches—the swaddling, the pacifier, the "lovey," the rocking and closeness with a parent—can act as helps in teaching the

baby an important mechanism—how to break the
cycle of intense, absorbing activity and give way
to sleep or to a restful, composed, quiet period.
When the child has developed his own inner
controls, the crutches gradually can be removed.

All children need to seek a goal and master it;
without such reward, little learning takes place
and there can be real frustration. As Dan grows
from infancy into childhood, his world must
include the opportunity for achievement, as well
as for fumbling and making mistakes. His mother
and father can provide tasks that are not too
difficult for him, and offer encouragement to
pursue a solution and praise when the end is
achieved. It will take time and patience for the
parents to do this, but it is certainly worthwhile.
Constantly chasing the child and interfering with
his activity not only will serve as a frustrating
inhibition, but also it is likely to provoke him to
more frantic behavior.

As Dan becomes excited after a success, he may
fall apart in a tantrum or a crying overreaction. I
would urge the parents to let him have his
tantrum or cry for a while, until his peak is
reached; then pick him up, gently but firmly
containing him, and sit down to rock and calm
him. This requires that they achieve control of
their own feelings.

It is hard not to join a child in a tantrum,
adding fuel to his fury. I have had to leave the
scene with my own children's tantrums in order
to gather my own composure, and then return to
pick them up and soothe them. If Dan's parents

can keep cool during his upsets, they can teach him how to control them for himself and then to bring himself down out of them. A child can learn these kinds of controls from his parents, just as he learns other things from them while he is growing up.

Every new task will be met with violent excitement as well as violent resistance. When Dan learns to feed himself, the floor may be covered with bits of food or his mouth may be stuffed with so much food that he chokes—unless some ingenious precautions are taken. Dan's mother will have to develop a rhythm for placing a few bits of food on Dan's tray at a time, supplying a few more as he needs them, rather than overwhelming him with a whole trayful. He would respond to being overwhelmed by overreacting, but if he can have only two pieces of food at once, swallow them, and then continue with more, he can master it. Dan's sense of achievement can be ample reward for his mother's patience.

More complex tasks, such as toilet training, are best postponed until Dan himself is ready for them. He would be easily frustrated and easily defeated if he were to fail, so there is less chance for setting up real problems if the timing can be geared to him. I would wait to introduce him to the pot until he is about two and a half—when he is beginning to want to imitate the other people in his environment and to organize things around him. Then as he is shown each step and encouraged to do it for himself, he can be led on to the next. If he can feel such a task as his own, the excitement will outweigh any resistance he might otherwise show. His second year will be fraught with incredible peaks of negativism anyway, and toilet training could be a real failure if it became a battleground.

Going to school can mean one of two things for a boy like Dan—he can find it an exciting outlet for all of his energy or he may be so frustrated by the necessary restrictions and so excited by the other children that he will fall apart.

A relaxed, easy nursery school that will let him learn how to get along with his peers and how to conform to the demands of a group can be a good first experience for Dan, and his mother will do well to prepare the way for him. First of all, she should talk with the teacher and enlist her understanding of the problem, and she should certainly stay with him the first few days of school. Preparing him ahead of time for the importance of trying to conform to the rules might help, and so will trying to cut down on extra pressure at home before and after school. Letting Dan know that she understands how hard it is for him to have to control himself for a period backs him up too.

The real problem with a boy like Dan is finding a way of supporting him without making him feel "different." He will see himself as odd and hopeless all too easily. Failures may pile up as he tries desperately to make a go of it with his peers and his teacher.

If Dan's parents can have achieved two things

by this time, they will be able to help him. They must have accepted him themselves, thereby learning to understand and enjoy him. And they must have learned to find a way of helping him face up to his own problems so that he feels a sense of mastery when he conquers them.

Relationships with other children can be hard for a boy like Dan. His parents can help by trying to arrange a one-to-one situation with other children, that is, one friend at a time. If he can make one good friend after school, this friend can help him into the group at school. The parents can foster such a friendship by taking the child on excursions with Dan.

Each new step of adjustment will be a hurdle for them all. The parents may need someone on whom they can rely for guidance and advice—and for letting off steam about their own feelings. If they are near either set of grandparents, this can be a help, but in most instances today young parents are alone and on their own. A sympathetic doctor or counselor may be a person to whom they can turn. In addition, in some localities parents of children like Dan, Matthew, and John are forming organizations through which they give one another emotional support and practical help. The growth of such groups is a direct expression of the number of people who have hyperactive children and who aren't content to "let them grow out of it."

It isn't easy to raise a child like Dan, Matthew, or John without becoming discouraged—but it is possible!

*The previous chapter won the 1973 Association for Children with Learning Disabilities Certificate of Merit after its appearance in* Redbook *magazine.*

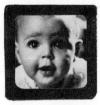 # Hyperactivity

No parent deserves more credit than do those of hyperactive children. These children demand more of their environment than they give back to it—and their demands are continuous—night and day. One of the most frustrating attributes of these children is that they are often very bright and attractive, and this fact constantly teases parents to feel that if they just had the right answers, if they had enough patience and the correct method, they could bring out the best in a child and suppress the worst side. Another difficulty is the kind of self-protective anger that these children's constant demands call up in an adult. And any parent is bound to feel guilty at being so angry with a small child. Since most of these children are highly sensitive to parental feelings, this excites them even more and their demands increase to a breaking point. The break is likely to be in the parents, for hyperkinesis has a kind of protective strength to it for the child. Parents say that even after they have learned to adjust to the constant, uncontrolled activity, they

worry about the child's future. And long before
school, they begin to worry about how such a
child will ever make it in a regimented learning
situation.

One of the most encouraging aspects of this
stressful condition is that the public has become
aware of how many of these children there are to
be incorporated into our society. I am sure that
their number has increased in recent years—in
part, due to the pressures of an intense,
uncompromising world. But along with this, the
recognition of this condition as one for which
society must take responsibility has helped
parents feel less lonely with it, less hopeless in
their efforts to prepare their thrashing,
hyperkinetic child for first grade. Special classes,
with more appropriate, person-to-person
supervision by specially trained teachers, are
being created in many schools. As I mentioned
earlier, parents' groups for desperate parents are
springing up, and, in them, parents can support
each other and can offer each other valuable
experience in handling these children. The
medical profession is beginning to recognize the
complexity of the problem—and are preparing
themselves with multidisciplined groups (of
physicians, social workers, psychologists,
therapists) to support and educate parents.

Presumably, with a multidisciplinary approach,
we can learn how to attack all aspects of the
problem at once: the child's hypersensitivity and
poorly organized neurological responses which are
reflected in the constant, frantic activity; the

parents' concerns and feelings of helplessness in the face of the battering they take in living with such a child; society's responsibility to accept these children as they are and to set up appropriate environments for teaching them how to live with themselves and others as well as how to learn. Learning can often become a very rewarding outlet for such children. To waste them as we have in the past would be a tragedy if society can do better. It will take a major reorganization of many of the resources we have for small children. Schools are set up for conformists, not individuals. One of the most dramatic examples of this came to my attention at a recent panel of educators, physicians, psychologists, and social scientists who met to consider the problem of hyperactive children in schools. It was reported that, on a sample check, 25 percent of the first-grade children in Harlem were being kept on drugs to keep them quiet in school. No one had thought to offer these children decent breakfasts which might have counteracted the hypoglycemia that made it impossible for many of these children to sit still. Drugs were an easier outlet and it kept alive the myth that these are damaged, second-rate children. And we are a chauvinistic society—especially when it comes to the point of dealing with difficult children.

The preceding article is an attempt to give parents of hyperkinetic children a new feeling of hopefulness, and certain practical means to prevent some of the future disturbed behavior and the consequent poor self-image in the child. One of the things that has helped me and the parents I have worked with has been the assurance that this condition can be dealt with preventively. The fact that there is a time in adolescence when these children will no longer be plagued by the problem of integrating their behavior is another reason for optimism. I hope that the sort of advice given here will help many families live through the initial difficult start to a brighter future.

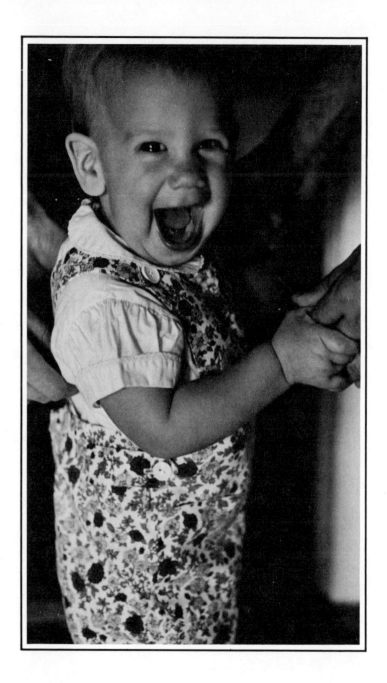

## Chapter 7

# How to set limits for toddlers

oon after a baby is able to explore and test the limits of everything around him or her, the parents are bound to ask their pediatrician a new type of question—"When do we start disciplining, and how?" A young mother brought her husband with her to my office to ask this question about their very active, determined little boy, ten-month-old Jamie, who was all over their three-room apartment. The week before he had found the garbage can, emptied the contents onto the kitchen floor, smeared tomato paste over his face, and begun to sputter over bits of meat and leftover spaghetti when his mother found him. She had remembered throwing away spoiled meat and called me to find out whether he could have poisoned himself by eating any of it. On another occasion he spilled soap powder all over the kitchen floor and then

proceeded to find and taste foot powder that his father had left beside his shoes. He ended up by turning on the bathtub faucets full blast and dropping in the stopper. Fortunately his aim with the stopper was not quite perfect and it had taken the tub awhile to fill, and this gave his parents time to discover what was happening.

His mother's account of a typical day was hilarious to hear, though poignant if one imagined what it was like for her. For she spent most of her time anticipating Jamie's next move and mopping up after his last one. Since his explorations were becoming more deliberate and many of them were potentially dangerous, his parents were frantic and had come to me for help.

Mr. Johnson blamed his wife for not "keeping an eye on Jamie," but freely admitted that he had been home on two occasions when Jamie was particularly uncontrollable and had not been able to stop him either. Mrs. Johnson was guilty, felt she had been neglectful and blamed herself for "spoiling" Jamie, for not being on the job every minute to prevent his escapades. At the same time she really could not see how she could stand any more from him.

"He makes me want to spank him," she said, "and I end up crying for being so angry with him. Should I spank him, or should I leave him in a playpen so he can't get into trouble? He just stands and screams if I do, and I can't bear that. But unless I follow him every minute, he finds some way to beat me. I stripped our house of traps and poisons, but he still finds new things. I'm afraid either he's going to kill himself or I'm going to kill him. What have I done wrong? How do we discipline him so he won't drive us all crazy?"

Mrs. Johnson was expressing what most mothers of active, inquisitive babies begin to feel at the end of the first year. The babies suddenly are free to explore a new, exciting world. They have mastered crawling and are in no mood to be stopped by a playpen or any other confinement. Since his mother had not started putting him in the playpen long enough ago for it to become a customary part of Jamie's day, it was not fair to expect him to accept it now.

The exploration and the crawling were such important achievements for the baby that the Johnsons knew they should take delight in them. And they did. They knew that Jamie was not "bad" when he got into things, and to punish him for natural, healthy progress seemed wrong. Yet they had to protect him from potential danger and try to maintain some kind of order in their home.

The problems that came with his progress were thus a source of real conflict for them: Jamie was undermining their self-confidence as parents and forcing them both to feel angry with themselves. This anger acted as a reinforcement to the anxiety that each of Jamie's escapades produced; indeed, the anxiety itself was so intense that the parents sought to rid themselves of it—by needing to hurt Jamie or punish him.

In order to help Mr. and Mrs. Johnson with this beginning crisis, I attempted to give them some

advice about Jamie and some understanding of
their own feelings. First of all, I told them that I
too would hate to curb Jamie through such drastic
measures as putting him in a playpen or in a safe
room alone. Therefore the house must be kept
babyproofed so that there wouldn't be anything
dangerous to get into. (Fortunately the peak periods
of exploration and testing do pass, and Jamie will
settle down for a while before the next peak period
comes—after he starts to walk.)

Then I told the Johnsons that since they knew
Jamie's behavior was normal, to treat it as if it was
a sign of being "spoiled" would be to miss the
point. This is not a matter for disciplinary
measures as such. One of the definitions of
discipline is "to bring under control." Jamie is not
out of control. The anxiety he causes in his parents
is out of control, and that is what needs to be
evaluated.

For instance, Mr. Johnson can take relief
responsibility more actively when he is home.
Perhaps he can even channel some of Jamie's
energy into more constructive forms of exploration.
He certainly can devise ways to babyproof cabinets
and drawers for his wife. But he also can support
rather than undermine his wife during the difficult
times.

During the next few months Mrs. Johnson's
patience will be tested repeatedly. A child Jamie's
age soon finds out, for instance, that he is not
supposed to play with the television set. As he
moves in on the fascinating array of dials and
buttons, he makes a noise or "happens" to call his

mother's attention to him, looking back at her expectantly and provocatively. If she removes him or tries to distract him, he *may* lose interest. But the chance is far greater that he will continue his game of teasing by returning to rattle the knobs and bang on the screen until he finally draws the response he is after—being stopped, definitely and firmly. If he is removed roughly but with conviction, the sensitive parent may well discern the child's relief and gratitude.

This relief points out the importance to a child of having someone in control at such a time. Somewhere inside, he knows he cannot stop himself, and he wants to be stopped. If there is no one to stop him, he must control himself—and that is infinitely harder and less fun.

Parents often ask me how their children will know the difference between the kinds of noes they must mete out in various situations. I assure them that children are geared to sort out important cues. And it is important to them as well as to the parents that the children learn when they mean business. The range or an electrical outlet, say, cannot be left in the teasing category with the television set or with Daddy's shirt drawer and Mother's workbox.

Parents, therefore, must decide which things are truly dangerous and then either babyproof these completely or, if that is impossible, make it absolutely clear that the child must *not* explore them. But if a child Jamie's age does not respond when his mother says, "No" to him about the oven door, for example, I would urge her to consider two

possibilities. Either she is saying, "No" to him so
frequently that it is losing meaning for him or she
isn't breaking through to him with enough of her
own conviction. If a simple no isn't enough, and
sometimes it may not be, I would not hesitate to
spank the child's hands or his bottom or to put him
in his bed. But I would *not* tease back and forth
about an important issue. Parents must take action
quickly and decisively.

Teaching a child discipline does not start with
the first sign of provocative behavior, although for
the parents it may seem to. Parents have been
teaching their children to set limits for themselves
from their earliest days. The way a mother protects
herself when a nursing baby bites her nipple, the
way a father firmly tucks a fussy baby into bed at
night, saying, "Now, go to sleep," each has
discipline in it.

The permissive era of the fifties demonstrated by
its mistakes that children longed for adults who
had their own convictions about limits and who
could pass them on. I remember in that period the
horror of watching a child disintegrate at the end
of a long day, building up anxiety, whirling around
provocatively, almost begging someone to say
firmly, "Now it is bedtime." When no one would,
he finally dissolved in screaming chaos until he
literally fell into bed by himself, exhausted.

Had his parents stopped or contained him, they
might have saved the child from this kind of ego
disintegration. Indeed, they could have taught him
the relief of learning limits for himself. Many
young parents I see today have been through this

formless kind of parenting with their own parents and are resolved not to repeat it with their children. I agree with them, for I think a parent's responsibility is to solidify the boundaries as well as the core of a child's ego. And boundaries protect as well as contain the more precious part of his or her personality.

Discipline can be built into a relationship with a child. Consideration, respect for family rules, acceptance of family duties—all can be natural results based on expectations of how people in a family will behave. Discipline is part of learning to live with others. In our society, however, it often is easier for parents to give in to their children's whims than it is to see the opportunity that's offered for teaching them social behavior. But if parents don't pass on their firm expectations about behavior, the children must spin their wheels more, waste precious energy searching for a "bedtime," find out the limits of danger for themselves. This is why I look upon the permissive era as anxiety-producing.

If Jamie continued to get himself into difficulties and be unresponsive to his mother when she said, "No," I would urge her to figure out where she stood on the issues of discipline. Through his behavior he may be saying to her that he knows she isn't very sure. It is good to resolve one's own ambivalence early about being a parent with authority, for there are stormier times ahead!

As the child grows a bit older his or her negativism increases, and so does the need for limits and discipline. But it may be harder for parents to distinguish their own problems with discipline from the child's. Let me present the problems of discipline with a slightly older child.

Mrs. Herman, a rather pretty, petite, tense young mother, cares a great deal about doing the right thing for her eighteen-month-old Eliza. Eliza is sturdy and rugged-looking like her father. Also like him, she looks up at her fluttering mother with a kind of tolerant stubbornness, which seems to be her response to Mrs. Herman's indecision.

Although Eliza was an easy baby, she was never gay or joyful, and I felt a certain amount of tension in the family. Mr. Herman left Eliza's care to his wife, "interfering as little as he possibly could." But he was sarcastic and scornful when things went wrong, and undermined his wife's shaky self-confidence in very subtle ways. From the beginning she turned to me for supportive advice, so I got to know her fairly well.

When I gave Eliza a shot at one year of age, the baby stuck out her lower lip. She gave her mother, who was holding her, an angry look and pushed her away instead of crying. This response to the shot was so telling in terms of their relationship and of the parents' tension that I made a note of it, and spoke to Mrs. Herman about it later.

With some relief she told me how inadequate and guilty she felt whenever anything went wrong with Eliza, and how frightened she was of being an inadequate mother for this child. She told me she had been a third daughter, and not a favored one, and had grown up afraid to assert herself. She had married her husband for his strong, silent qualities, hoping that he could compensate for what she felt she lacked. Until Eliza came, their marriage had been a good one, and each had indeed found the other a complementary partner.

But Eliza had been wanted so much that her very importance had come between them. They began to quarrel, and Eliza seemed to grow more and more like her father. Now every time anything went wrong, both Eliza and her father seemed to look at Mrs. Herman with the same kind of reproach for her incompetence. Indeed, I had seen the devastating strength of such a look from Eliza, so I could understand her mother's feelings.

At eighteen months Eliza was becoming a real problem. She was demanding of her mother, whimpering or crawling up and down in her lap when Mrs. Herman tried to talk to me. When her mother tried to ignore her, Eliza began to unload the diaper can, to tear the magazines in my office, to open the drawers that contained medicines. Her mother seemed helpless in the face of these assaults.

I told Eliza that I knew she did not want her mother to talk to me, but that we were going to continue and that I expected her to leave my things alone and play with the many toys there for her. She looked up at me defiantly, obviously taking in my reprimand. Angrily she lay down on the floor and began to kick and thrash, screaming at the top of her voice. Her mother rushed to her side and fluttered around her, trying alternately to distract, to cajole, and to pet her. Her mother's efforts added fuel to Eliza's tantrum, and she kicked her mother as she hovered above her. Mrs. Herman looked helpless at first, then angrily she looked up at me and shouted, "Now see what you've done! Now she'll never let you examine her. It serves you right!"

I felt this was a pretty important time to help mother and daughter with their rather tense relationship. I do not feel that temper tantrums are at all unusual or abnormal in the second year. Eliza's response to being frustrated by me was an expectable and even healthy one. But I did not feel it presaged very well for her future development that her mother felt so helpless and so guilty that she must descend to Eliza's two-year-old level, even to the extent of having a tantrum with her.

There was probably nothing Mrs. Herman could have done to stop Eliza's tantrum, nor did she need to stop her. The tantrum was serving its own purpose. Still, the kind of inner turmoil that tantrums represent demand strength in adults around a two-year-old. Mrs. Herman was caught up in her own feelings and was in no way helping Eliza with hers. After "their" tantrum was over, I urged Mrs. Herman to think with me about the family's relationships and added, "If you don't have discipline problems already with Eliza, you soon will have." Mrs. Herman behaved as if I had opened a box of magic. Her eyes widened in surprise; she looked at me and said, "How did you know?"

I assured her it was an inevitable part of the second year for children to push parents to their limits. And since I was pretty sure Eliza knew how inadequate she made her mother feel whenever things went wrong, I could assume that this would be a rough period for them. Mrs. Herman began to tell me about some of their bad times.

Eliza defied her openly, even dangerously, by getting into forbidden activities. On occasion she had run out into the street, despite her mother's orders. She whined continually when they were alone together, asking to be picked up, then put down, screaming with indecision or frustration at every turn. Her mother tried to please her in every way but seemed unable to find out or provide what she wanted. She offered her cookies and candy, but Eliza threw them on the rug and ground them with her foot. When her mother tried to talk on the phone, Eliza would climb into her lap, grab for the phone and scream into it until Mrs. Herman had to hang up.

When Mr. Herman came home at night, Eliza demanded and received all his attention, even taking him off into a room with her alone. No one seemed able to say no to her, and Mr. Herman blamed his wife openly for the child's frantic discontent. Mrs. Herman blamed herself too, but she was at a loss as to how to handle it. She expected me to tell her to put her foot down and discipline Eliza, but she knew she couldn't do that, so she didn't even want to hear me say it.

Mrs. Herman was right in part. Eliza's "spoiled" behavior had created a strong reaction in me of wanting to punish her, to stop her, or to shut her up. I think this is a universal reaction that such behavior in children calls forth from adults. And by the same token it is a cry for help from the child. Indeed, I think he or she is asking for limits from a caring adult. But the limits must be part of the adult's total commitment to the child, not just a reaction to the immediate, provoking behavior. In this case I was more concerned with what Eliza's cry for help was based upon—tension between the parents, the mother's loss of self-confidence, the kind of hostility toward Eliza that had built up as a result of Mrs. Herman's feelings of helplessness.

In order for Mrs. Herman to be able to offer Eliza the kind of discipline that might work, she needed to overcome her own indecision, her own angry feelings; and at the same time she needed to realize that it was important for Eliza to have a parent who was understanding but also firm, who could not be pushed around by her two-year-old negativism.

As we talked about the underlying reasons for their difficulties with discipline, Mrs. Herman began to be able to see that it wasn't so much what she did to discipline or contain Eliza as it was that Eliza needed conviction from her mother as to limits as much as she needed other signs of caring. And as she began to understand Eliza's needs as a two-year-old, Mrs. Herman began to gather confidence.

At the end of our session, after we had agreed that the next step was to get Mr. Herman to come in for a family session, Mrs. Herman said firmly but pleasantly to Eliza, "Now it's time for Dr. Brazelton to examine you. Sit here in my lap so I

can show you what he will do. I think you'll even
like it."

Eliza was so surprised at her mother's new tone
that she submitted to being undressed. She sat in
her mother's lap, protested my passes at her a few
times, but seemed to understand that her mother
and I were both united and firm about completing
the exam. She listened and watched when I
showed her how the stethoscope worked and how I
would examine her with it.

At the end of the very successful examination, I
congratulated Eliza and gave her a toy as a reward.
She danced gaily around my room as if she had
really mastered a big step. As I congratulated her
mother on her own mastery, I pointed out that this
kind of firm, understanding expectation had meant
a great deal to Eliza.

I am reminded of this family when parents ask
me what kind of discipline to use when their
children need to be punished. Should they try
reasoning with them, isolating them, putting them
in their bed or their room? Should they try to
distract them or show they are disappointed in
them? Should they speak sharply or resort to a slap
or spanking?

There isn't just one answer. The discipline
should fit the child and it should fit the crime—but
above all it should be accompanied by a conviction
on the parents' part that setting limits is an
important aspect of caring for small children. And
unless this sense of caring accompanies discipline,
discipline remains *just* punishment. The goal of
discipline is to help the child learn his own limits

and eventually find the relief of having inner discipline built into his capacity for living a full, rich, and considerate life.

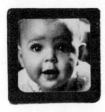

# Discipline

There are sociological reasons why discipline is such an issue in this generation. The swing away from discipline in the forties and fifties has provided us with a discontented, angry generation who will tell you that one of the hardest aspects of growing up for them was that their parents never helped them learn self-limits. One eighteen-year-old girl told me that she looks back on her childhood as a nightmare of indecision, and she feels that her parents "copped out," didn't care what she did. Another reason is that parents today are insecure and fear doing something wrong; discipline is so hard for parents that it quickly becomes an area they would rather leave to the child. The guilt one suffers after effectively reprimanding a small child is instinctive, and inevitable. A third factor is becoming more and more of a public one—the possibility of child abuse. Every parent feels that he or she might hurt a child while angry. And indeed one occasionally does. Hence, the overreaction which a parent feels before driven to discipline a child becomes a counter to effective discipline. We are all afraid

(and appropriately) of really expressing our
feelings toward a naughty, demanding toddler.

But as I have pointed out in the preceding
article, it is very important to small children to
have limits established by the environment which
are firm, reliable, and reassuring. One needs only
to watch an anguished two-year-old in a severe
temper tantrum to recognize the lengths to which
his or her inner turmoil will lead. And the
provocative behavior of a "spoiled child," which
drives every adult to feel that he or she should say
"No" to the child, is another indication of the
power behind the toddler's need for limits. The
relief one sees in the child's eyes when an adult
says, "Stop that or I'll stop you!" is indicative of
what drives the child on to provoking behavior. So
—the need is there in the child.

When should discipline start? In my opinion it
should start when children begin to indicate that
this is what they need. At the end of the first year,
a crawling baby will crawl up to a forbidden
television set or light plug, turn slyly around to be
sure a parent is watching—then continue to tease
until he or she has provoked the parent to react.
Parents try distraction. They remove as many of
the offending situations as they can. They say "No"
firmly. But the child persists in this rather
dangerous behavior. At this point, discipline *that
works* must take over. Either firm removal to
another room, or a spanked hand, or whatever is
necessary to settle the issue could be the answer to
the child's demands at the time. Each parent must
gauge the particular method of discipline to his or

her own responses and to what works for the child.

Certainly, discipline should be used sparingly. Constant nagging prohibitions soon become meaningless, or, worse, they keep the child under such a negative cloud of pressure that the whole personality must suffer. Certainly physical punishment should be used as little as possible and as a last resort—but it may well be necessary to clear the air. The most difficult and ill-advised use of discipline that I know of is to postpone it and to keep it as an ax hanging over the child's head. "Daddy will punish you when he gets home! Just wait till we get to the car—and you'll get it! I have to get over my anger before I can punish you, but we'll have a long talk about it then." Postponed discipline becomes something else—it becomes vindictive and destructive. Immediately administered discipline has a different value—it is directly associated with the forbidden or dangerous act.

The problem for most of the present generation of parents is that they have never had experience with a secure kind of discipline. Most of us who were parents at the time these young people were growing up were full of conflict about whether to set limits or not. There was a powerful trend to let children's individuality express itself—a feeling that eventually they would find limits for themselves, and they would be "theirs" rather than "ours." That hasn't worked for all the reasons we've mentioned. Any society needs to impose limits on individuality to protect the needs of others, and ours has proved to be no exception. So parents must get on with the job of providing a more secure base for the next generation. It may well be a period of rather tortured exploration, but understanding the child's needs and watching for cues from him or her may help determine the course.

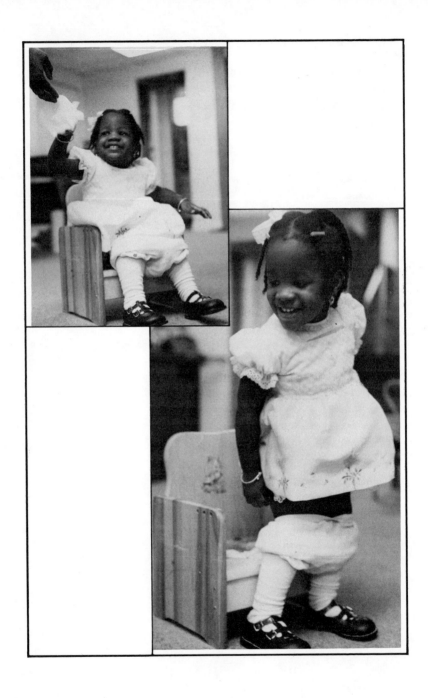

## Chapter 8

# Toilet training: a step-by-step approach

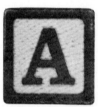tall, willowy brunette with a British accent brought her eighteen-month-old Sarah to my office for a checkup recently. Sarah was a very active little girl. She rapidly cased my office with her eyes as she entered. As soon as they came through the door, she squirmed out of her mother's arms, hitting the floor, with a bang. She gathered herself up and crossed the room in a split second, leaning forward at an angle to walk in such a hurry that I worried whether she would be able to stop. She adroitly leaned backward as she got to the toy chest, pulling herself up to a sudden stop from her rapid forward motion. So sudden was it that she flopped backward into a sitting position— as if this was what she had planned. She proceeded to take out, examine, and discard each of the twenty-five toys in the chest. I had just had time to ask her mother how the two of them were

when Sarah was up and away, my desk her next
goal.

I successfully headed her off, but aimed her in
the direction of my bookcase without realizing my
mistake. Before Mrs. Stewart could answer my
initial question, Sarah had stripped my bookcase
of its contents and was headed for my desk again.
The rest of our interview was spent in keeping
her away from my files, allowing her to climb up
and over me and the desk, offering her toys,
which she refused. Finally I gave up the notion of
interviewing her mother to concentrate on playing
with Sarah as I examined her. And that was fun!

She was not fearful. She was delighted with
each maneuver I made as long as she could
participate in it. She allowed me to poke into her
ears and her throat as long as she could poke into
mine. When it came time to weigh her, she
bounced up and down on the scales fearlessly and
then quickly imitated me after I showed her how
to stand still. I had to assume a stiff, stylized
position, legs wide apart, in order to capture her
interest. But she picked up the humor of my
posture and copied it for my approval.

After this exciting performance, I was Sarah's
slave. Soon I was down on the floor with her,
playing with blocks and talking to her mother as
we played. Mrs. Stewart began to tell me the story
of Sarah's toilet training, and she spoke as if she
was now in a hopeless, losing struggle. She had
started training Sarah at six months, according to
her own mother's written instructions from
England. She had sat Sarah on a pot in her lap

after each meal and when she picked her up from sleep.

Sarah had been active from the first, and it was difficult to make her sit still very long, but Mrs. Stewart was determined. Very quickly Sarah seemed to sense that it was easier to comply, for after that she was given her freedom to explore, to play with her mother, or to be rewarded with a "sweet." From the way Mrs. Stewart described this period, I am sure Sarah also sensed that her mother's tension would evaporate only after they both had succeeded.

The training seemed to be a success, and Sarah was dry for most of the day and occasionally had her bowel movements on the potty as well. Her grandmothers in England were delighted. But Mrs. Stewart had noticed that Sarah's bowel patterns changed when she was about a year old, and she began to be constipated more often. Despite laxative foods, Sarah seemed to be straining at times during the day, but did not produce what her mother expected. When she did have a movement, she seemed to save it for nighttime and her diapers. As if this wasn't bad enough, now Sarah seemed to be holding onto her urine as well.

She refused to perform on the potty that her mother provided after meals and before bedtime, and she almost defiantly wet her pants and the floor as soon as she managed to escape from the pot. Her mother had tried strapping her onto it, had spanked her or put her to bed. Nothing worked, and Sarah's defiance was stronger, her

negative behavior toward training more and
more upsetting. She was smearing her bowel
movements over her bed, wetting the floor
willfully in front of her mother's friends and
when her father came home at night. And Mrs.
Stewart's main concern was that her own mother
was coming soon from England—to catch them in
this terrible failure!

As she told me this her voice began to break.
Sarah had been playing with toys across the room,
but as she heard her mother's change in tone, she
turned and sped over to her. She climbed up in
her lap, cuddled against her, put her thumb in
her own mouth, laid her other hand gently on her
mother's, and sat quietly for the rest of our time
together.

This complete change in Sarah was the most
remarkable piece of behavior I had seen. She had
sensed her mother's despair. Year-and-a-half-old
Sarah essentially was mothering her mother!

Do you see the strengths in this child as I do?
She was telling her mother in definite, clear
behavioral messages that their conflict was an
unnecessary one. Sarah was too strong and too
determined to have things done to her. Although
she had gone along with her mother's demands
for toilet training in the first year, since that
made it easier to get on to the more exciting
rewards of her day, it could not last. As the desire
for independent activity and freedom to make her
own choices became more important in the
second year, Sarah began to indicate that she was
no longer willing to comply.

If she were a less determined little person, the

punishment and disapproval would have succeeded, and Sarah might have shoved this conflict down under the surface. I am sure that this is what happens to many children who appear to give in to their parents' pressure to conform. In fact, children who comply too easily worry me, because I wonder where and when their need to sort out their ambivalence about being dependent will surface.

It doesn't surprise me when this conflict shows up in bed-wetting or in bowel difficulties when the child is older. For example, there is a report that among draftees in England 15 percent of the eighteen-year-olds are bed-wetters!

The negativism and defiance that came to the surface in Sarah's second year are important to her independence. At this age she needed to walk, to run, to be on the go. To be set down to do passively what her mother required of her was not likely to produce success. Sarah had to be shown the steps to such a complex task as toilet training in a way that would make them interesting to her and worth her imitation. She certainly had the incentive to imitate, but she needed to do it on her own.

With this in mind, I was able to comfort Mrs. Stewart about her fears of failure as a mother, and I urged her to reconsider her own determination to "train" Sarah. We both knew Sarah knew what was expected of her, and I was sure that sooner or later she would want to please her mother again.

Mrs. Stewart was able to listen and to believe in my understanding of Sarah's strengths, for somewhere she felt them too. When they got home, she put Sarah back in diapers, telling her it was all right for her to be in them. She had her mother telephone me when they hit the expected snag shortly after her arrival, and I explained our reasoning.

The depth of Sarah's intuition is expressed in a final event: Within a week after her grandmother went home and at the age of twenty-one months, Sarah trained herself completely—day and night!

The problems that result from a rigid method of toilet training are often difficult to remedy afterward, and I would not have predicted such early success for Sarah and her mother after a conflict of this dimension had been set up. If Mrs. Stewart and I had discussed this in advance, I would have urged a program of training that tries to avoid problems.

My program consists of a number of steps designed to encourage children to train themselves *at their own speed*. I urge mothers—and fathers, even grandparents—to wait until the last half of the second year and until the child demonstrates a kind of readiness.

You might tell that your child is ready for toilet training if he behaves in any of the following ways: (1) He is over the excitement of just having learned to walk and run and is able to sit down quietly to play for a period. (2) He demonstrates an interest in the toilet and what it is used for. (3) He shows imitative behaviors, such as brushing his teeth or "shaving" or setting the table or mopping up spilled food and drink. (4) He is able to understand and participate in discussions about "feeling the need to go" and why it might be desirable to do something as difficult as holding on to his urine or stool and then going to a special place to perform. (5) He shows strong evidence of wanting to put his toys or his clothes where they belong; indeed, he may be almost compulsive about this. (6) He is not in a violently negative period—that is, he will not explode in a tantrum when you suggest that he do something.

Once you have decided that your child is ready to begin training, here are some methods you might follow:

1. Place a potty chair on the floor in the bathroom and tell him it is his own. Once a day take him to sit on it for a short period *in his clothes.* You might sit on the "adult" toilet and read to the child, give him a cookie, or use any appropriate incentive to make it worth his while. A short period of sitting is all that is necessary to institute this routine, and you must *not* restrain him if he wants to leave. Toilet training must be thought of as a ritual in which he himself wants to participate.

He will not like the feeling of the pot if he is undressed initially. If he performs on it early in this period, it may frighten him, and he may not be willing to perform again for months. Children do see their urine and bowel movements as part of themselves—even precious parts of themselves. I have never been convinced that babies are uncomfortable instinctively when they are wet or dirty. I think that revulsion and discomfort are

built in from the outside and cannot be depended
on to be a force for a child's wanting to be
trained.

2. After he is accustomed to the daily ritual and
has accepted it as his own, take him to sit on the
pot without his clothes and diapers. Aim for a
time when he is likely to have a bowel movement
—it is best for him to realize what he is doing
when he begins to perform.

3. Continue the routine time on the pot for about
a week. In addition, take him to his toilet to sit
down right after he has had a bowel movement in
his diapers. Undo his dirty diaper and let him see
what it is that you have been wanting of him. You
can say that Mother and Dad go to sit on their pot
and that he has his own, and someday he will use
it as they do.

At this stage do not take his dirty diaper away
immediately to flush his stool down the toilet.
Wait until he loses interest. Although he may
seem intrigued with watching his bowel
movement flush away, many children express
fears later on which show that they have been
frightened. You are building up his desire to give
up this part of himself—don't push it too fast!

4. If he begins to be interested and cooperative,
take him several times a day to the potty to see if
he is willing to be "caught" when he indicates he
is ready to urinate or have a movement.

If he allows himself to be caught, for example,
after a meal or during a bath or when he is dry,
praise him—but don't overdo it. You can turn a
child off all too easily with too much praise in the
second year and in this negative period. The

highest praise may be to say he's just like an
older brother or sister whom he knows is trained.
Allowing him to watch a child his own age
perform on the pot may be the best incentive.

5. When you are sure he is ready, allow him to
play for periods without any clothes on from the
waist down. Put the pot in his room or in the yard
with him. Tell him that this is done so that he
can take over the whole process. Offer to remind
him periodically to try to perform. Then, *if* he is
not resistant, remind him hourly that he might
want to go himself. If his interest lags or if he
shows any resistance or if he has an accident, do
not press this step. Put him back in diapers and
wait. He will tell you in some way when he is
ready.

In a series of 1170 children whose mothers tried
this method and kept records, 940 trained
themselves for bowel and bladder simultaneously
and accomplished it almost overnight. The
average age for this initial success was 27.7
months.

6. After he wants to control himself and can do
it, put him in training pants, which he can pull
down himself. If you try these too soon, they do
not help—they feel too much like his accustomed
diapers, and he wets without thinking. As a result
he may be so pressed by embarrassment or a
sense of failure that he may give up the effort.

7. Many children, especially boys, who train
themselves for urinating begin to hold back on
their bowel movements. I think this means that
the youngster is not quite ready to give in to all of
society's demands about his bathroom habits.

Further, a child sees his bowel movements as a more tangible part of himself than his urine, so it takes greater effort for him to give them up. Don't urge or cajole him. If you do, he may easily get into a vicious circle of holding back his stools, becoming constipated, hurting himself with a hard stool, and creating an anal fissure; then constipation becomes a physical as well as a psychologically complicated situation.

If constipation does seem to be a problem, give your child laxative foods or stool softeners. Reassure him that it is perfectly all right to save his bowel movement for a time when he's diapered, and provide him with diapers at such times as a naptime and nighttime.

8. Standing up to urinate is an exciting step for a boy. He had better learn it after he has learned to sit for his bowel movements, for it is so much fun for him to stand and spray into the toilet that he won't be willing to sit down again after he learns it. He will learn by watching his father or another little boy.

While he is still sitting on his potty seat to urinate, I would never use the guards that are provided for boys to prevent their wetting the floor. Sooner or later this guard will hurt him as he is getting on or off the toilet seat, and he will become reluctant to sit down again. Moreover, a boy quickly learns to hold his penis down in order to make noise in the pot with his urine.

9. Nap and night training should be left until well after the child has been clean and dry for a long period. (This advice also applies to taking the child with you when you go shopping or visiting—

keep him in diapers until both of you are *sure* he can make it without them.) He can usually be depended on to voice an interest in giving up his diapers at night, so don't press him until he is ready.

If he "sleeps too hard" or is resistant to being awakened to go or any of the many other excuses I hear, it simply means he is not at the point of feeling the urge to be this mature. For this reason I do not recommend the use of gadgets that waken a child as soon as he wets himself or pills that keep him dry. Such devices are aimed at the symptom. Unless they are used carefully and coupled with a child's real desire to achieve night control, they may reinforce his despair and act as a kind of punishment when he fails.

When a child is ready and wants to be helped to stay dry at night, I would urge that you discuss it with him in the evening before bedtime. Then before you yourself go to bed, wake him and see if he is willing to get himself up to go to the toilet. (Carrying him to the bathroom while he is asleep doesn't really help, and it is not likely to engender the kind of mastery that he needs to achieve control by himself.) If he can do this himself, he also can begin to get himself up in the early morning to urinate when he needs to. You may help him by putting his pot, painted with luminous paint, by the bed. Then he can see it when you get him up.

As soon as he is ready to take over by himself, I would make it as easy for him as you can with such gadgets as a night light or a luminous clock. Staying dry all night is a very big step in the process of maturation, and a very important one to a child's self-image. As long as he wets himself at night, he sees himself as immature and inadequate. Helping him with these feelings is the important job—not pushing him, or punishing him if he doesn't stay dry.

These nine steps merely outline the role of a parent as a helper in a child's *own* progress toward maturity.

In the study of 1170 children mentioned earlier, there were only 16 (1.5 percent) who were still wetting the bed after five years of age. On the average, daytime training had been completed by the age of 28 months; and in 80 percent of the cases, night training was done by the age of three. Boys took 2.5 months longer to complete training than girls, and first children were delayed 1.7 months in relation to their siblings.

The best thing about toilet training is that when it is done successfully, everybody can forget about it.

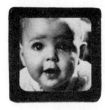

# Leaving it up to the child

In the past twenty years of my practice as a pediatrician, I have seen toilet training change from a major problem in childrearing to a minor one. No longer are pediatric clinics filled with bed-wetters. Chronic constipation and soiling are much rarer symptoms of stress in school-age children. Young mothers are not so vulnerable to grandparents' accusations of neglect if they have not followed the European tradition of training their baby by the end of the first year—as soon as his or her reflex controls make it possible. Even ten years ago, a mother might feel herself a failure if her child lagged behind her neighbor's in getting trained in the second year. Now a two-and-a-half-year-old who is still in diapers is not a cause for uptight concern. The language of young parents has changed from "I haven't got him trained" to "He isn't ready to train himself yet." This is a remarkable transition.

What has happened? I think that we have begun to see toilet training in its proper light—a developmental step that children want to achieve for themselves as they build toward their own strong, vital personalities. In this country, we have begun to give young children more credit for their strengths—and one of these strengths is that even when they are little they want to please those around them and to adapt to society's requirements. Children want to attain a more grown-up status—and many parents now realize that they don't have to press their children into conforming to adult expectations, to "housebreak" them *before* they are old enough to rebel. In fact, the intensity of a two-year-old's desire to imitate older children, or his or her own-age peers and even the adults around has always surprised me. The sensitivity of children of this age to the tasks which are required of them to become adults is remarkable. At a time when they appear to be negative most of the time, when any request from their parents meets with an automatic "No," they seem to be able to master complex behavioral steps *on their own.* They try to brush their teeth, shave like father, put on pieces of clothing. And it is no coincidence that this is a time when they can be captured to conform to society's rules about toileting.

Training children in other cultures has interested me, for it does not appear to be the problem that we tend to create in ours. In Mexico and in Africa, where children are carried on their mothers' backs, diapers are discontinued after a few months. The mother (or caretaker) is in constant contact and holds the infant away from her to urinate or to produce a bowel movement whenever she gets an appropriate signal. Mothers there have told me that a baby's belly tightens just prior to urinating or defecating. When children can walk, they quickly learn to step outside the hut to the nearby cornfield. When they make a mistake inside the hut, they are mildly reproved, but I have never seen a toddler punished for mistakes in the area of toileting. In fact, the commonest reaction is that of laughter and a comment, "He's too little to know better." Since, in the cultures that I have studied, there is an underlying emphasis on growing up rapidly to assume an adult role, it is not surprising that even a small child wants to imitate adults. As our culture became more "civilized" (and more compulsively clean and structured), we have been through a period of strict and punitive approaches to cleanliness, orderliness, and to toilet training in infancy which seemed to many of us in pediatrics to be counterproductive. A high incidence of enuresis, chronic constipation which can last into adulthood, and soiling or smearing with feces by four- and five-year-old children are problems that seem to be all too common in our Western cultures. These end results have always seemed to me to be rather expectable as symptoms from rebellious children whose need for autonomy in these areas has not been recognized.

Once I became aware of this, I tried to determine the stage at which a child's own developmental processes became ready to master the requirements of our complicated society. To recognize the urge to urinate or defecate, to realize that one must retain it, and to get to and deposit urine or feces in a special place designated by adults is a lot to expect of a small child. But we do see toddlers master this complex series of expectations in less complex societies, and this led me to wonder how to construct a framework for young mothers which would work in our own. The suggestions in the preceding article were the result. However, since we have been burdened for so long with the idea that children must *be trained,* many young mothers will continue to feel that it is their "job" to train their children. Even when society is changing its attitude to a more child-oriented developmental approach, young mothers can still be made to feel guilty if their child has not achieved this step as early as the neighbor's child. It may take a generation or two of children who are successful in training themselves before the majority of parents can believe it possible to leave it to them.

But in time, I am sure we can convince young parents that it is better to allow the child to achieve toilet training as he or she does any other developmental step—with all the excitement of mastery, and the ego reinforcement that each new step can bring.

Left entirely to their own devices and without any outside help, children ultimately would manage to train themselves successfully. The parents' role is simply to make the children's job easier, to suggest the idea but allow them to master it on their own, and at their own speed. Once you have followed the steps outlined in the preceding section, your job is done. Having made certain that your child has understood these steps, as well as your desire to see them accomplished, you must get out of the picture. You have done your part in showing the child what is expected. If you keep pressing the child to perform or even reminding him or her, you are putting on pressure. And it *will* be counterproductive. We have said that toilet training should be an autonomous step or it is likely to fail. Don't act as if you are turning the situation over to the child, but then sit over him or her with "kindly" insistence, demanding conformity without regard for your child's own pattern. There are too many and too individualized reasons why a particular child may not want to grow up, to be like others in this area. And they aren't all irrevocable ones, by any means. They become irrevocable when they are made into a battleground by parents who feel they *must* succeed. Our last child continued to wet his bed until he had passed the age when I thought it was normal. I got him up each morning and silently but grimly helped him change his bed. One morning, he sighed and said, "I wish you didn't care so much, Dad." I quickly denied that it mattered a bit to me, but I realized he was right. I stopped caring "so much" and he stopped wetting. A rare coincidence, indeed!

But how can one stop caring, when all of the neighbors' children of similar age are trained? When grandparents start their weekly calls with, "Hasn't she performed *yet?*" When you *know* the child knows what to do and is smart enough to do it. Should he or she be punished, for you know that would do the trick? Since it is a defiant act, shouldn't it be met with discipline?

I can almost promise that a disciplinary approach will fail, for it places toilet training in a target area—a target for regression whenever the child feels under pressure later on, or whenever he or she is angry with you or is unhappy or lonely. Do you really want to set it up that way? Is the battle that important? To balance this, the children who wait until their own timing for performance is met are the ones who literally train themselves overnight—and they accomplish day and night training all at once. For it's *their* achievement. This is well worth waiting for. This is no place for a battle. Feeding and toileting are areas that are too important to most children, and they will win any battle set up by parents in these areas.

*What age should one begin to worry?*

Until three and a half or four years of age, I think
it can be normal for a child to want to resist adult
demands in the area of daytime training. Beyond
that, I would wonder why he or she wasn't more
interested in growing up. For this kind of
compliance is expected by peers, by everyone
around. Nursery school conversations between
three- and four-year-olds are loaded with
questions (and pressure) about toilet training.
When four-year-olds are still wetting and soiling, I
would begin to assess their lives for too much
outside pressure, or for other reasons why they
are unable or unwilling to want to get daytime
trained.

*Enuresis*

I do not feel that wetting the bed should be taken
as seriously at these ages. Many children want to
control themselves at night, just as they do in the
daytime, but cannot control themselves over an
eight- to twelve-hour stretch until the ages of six
or seven. As long as they don't feel inadequate or
guilty, I think it can and should be looked upon as
an individual difference in timing. Parents often
apologetically say that their child is too heavy a
sleeper, or has too small a bladder, or too little
control. These may all be individual differences in
many children and may contribute to difficulty in
gaining night control. I'm sure that pressure from
the environment, or from within the child (when

he or she feels like a failure) will complicate this situation. So I would certainly urge parents against shaming a child or allowing him or her to feel guilty for this. Again, many parents say, "He doesn't seem to notice or care," and they feel they must enforce discipline to press the child to care. In the first place, I don't believe that a child doesn't care, and I would rather suspect that he or she cared too much. So an understanding, helpful, unpressured approach which reinforces the child's own feelings of adequacy and of wanting to grow up is much more effective.

If the *child* wants you to help, you can offer to get him or her up before you go to bed. You can put a special pot by the bedside, as a symbol of your desire to help. When you rouse the child to get up, by *himself* or *herself,* he or she can be taught to urinate into this pot. Then the child can more easily roll out of bed in the early morning to this available pot. But all of these maneuvers can add more pressure and more feelings of failure to an already defeated child if they are not seen as helpful to his or her *own* efforts.

### Constipation

One of the commonest reasons for small children's holding back bowel movements can come from their own burning desire to get themselves trained. I have often heard parents describe a toddler who is already urinating in the toilet, and who is terribly proud of his or her newfound achievement, but who hides in a corner to defecate. Other children howl with pain or

anguish as they feel a bowel movement coming.
Parents report that they must be in pain and
make the mistake of manipulating them with
suppositories or enemas "to relieve them." I think
they are often caught in their own ambivalence
about letting go of all of these controls. Having
made a big step in giving up their urine to the
toilet, they are *unconsciously* unable to make the
next step. And, as in other areas in the second and
third years, they get so tortured about making a
decision that they force themselves into an
internal struggle. This struggle has its problems,
for the harder they try to resolve this inner
conflict, the more they succeed in tightening up.
And constipation may well result. As they hold
back their stools, they indeed become constipated.
The hard movement that results hurts them when
they finally do perform, and it becomes a physical
holding back as well. For when the anal sphincter
has been fissured by a rocky movement, it will go
into reflex spasm for each succeeding movement.
At this point, it is a vicious cycle—physical as
well as psychological—and chronic constipation
can follow.

Before this becomes a fixed pattern, I would
urge a double approach: (1) Get the advice of your
physician. Use stool softeners and natural or mild
laxatives which you can use safely for a
prolonged period. When you have been successful
in softening the stools, be sure you continue, and
then you can begin to reassure the child (and the
sphincter) that the bowel movements will no
longer hurt. (2) Take any pressure off the child to
perform. If he or she is caught up in a struggle

about where to have a BM, say that the diaper is especially for this. Reassure the child that it is not important where the bowel movement takes place, and try to help him or her relax at such a time. Offer a quiet place to hide or lie down, and assure the child that it is *his* or *her* choice, not yours. I would also be sure that you avoid other sources of pressure for a while—siblings who tease, peers or teachers who expect success, grandparents who shame. This is a time for reassurance and the comfort of being understood and protected. For it can build up into a pretty painful, horrendous situation for everyone.

If, in spite of following this advice, a problem has arisen and you cannot resolve it alone, do seek professional help for yourself and your child before he or she begins to feel like a failure and an inadequate person. I'm sure that many adults who put themselves down at every turn can trace the early beginning of a poor self-image to their "failures" in achieving autonomy in the area of toilet training.

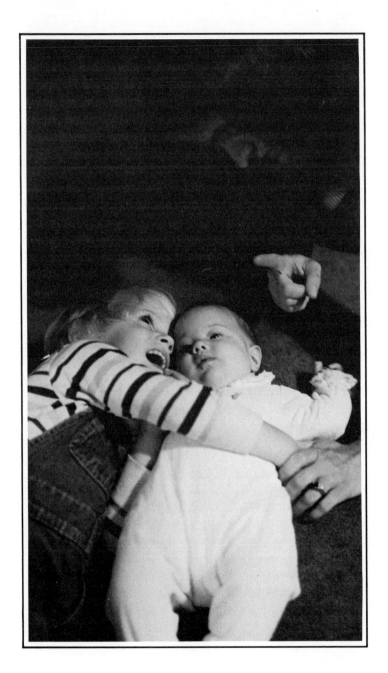

## Chapter 9

# The case for sibling rivalry

*May 4*

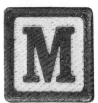rs. Shaw brought Tom into my office at the age of eighteen months for his periodic checkup. Mrs. Shaw is a pretty woman, and usually impeccably groomed. Today she looked distraught and tired and carelessly put together. After we had talked about Tom's health and physical development, I asked her whether she was having any problems with him. I got more than I had bargained for.

"He collapses on the floor when I ask him to do anything! He screams at me when I try to stop him from throwing food around the kitchen or when I tell him he mustn't touch the hot stove. He seems to be testing me at every turn, and I just feel like having a tantrum with him. In fact, I do sometimes scream back at him—which just makes him laugh. He's a monster, all of a sudden!"

Since this seemed to me to be fairly standard behavior for an eighteen-month-old (a surge of negativism occurs in most babies at some point in the second year), I was not prepared for the weeping that followed Mrs. Shaw's outburst. I had tagged her as a controlled, organized mother who cared deeply about Tom and had created a warm, loving environment for her outgoing little boy.

Tom was active and aggressively inquisitive, but he also seemed very aware of adults and what they expected of him. He churned around my office, examining every object in it, watching me out of the corner of his eye, and then bringing a toy for my approval in an attempt to include me in his gay excitement. One couldn't help but enjoy Tom and admire him and his mother.

After Mrs. Shaw's tears subsided, I asked why Tom's behavior upset her so much. I had assured her on a previous visit that this kind of negativism was to be expected and was perfectly normal even if it wasn't easy to live with. I reminded her that at the time she had even expressed some delight in Tom's stubbornness and boyish badness.

"But since then things have changed between us, and Tommy knows it," she told me. "Now he just does these things to torture me. I get so angry that I'm afraid I won't love him at all!"

I showed my surprise and she blurted out, "But you see, I'm pregnant! I've deserted Tommy and he knows it. I feel so bad for him—and for me too. If I didn't think it was hard on a child to be the only child in a family, I'd have been tempted not to have another. It was perfect just as it was. I know I can never feel the same about another baby as I do about Tommy. I don't feel that I can mother two babies without cheating them both."

Mrs. Shaw was expressing a feeling common to most mothers when they face a second pregnancy. The more a woman cares for her first child and the more she wants to do an "ideal" job with him, the more anguish she is likely to feel about "deserting" him and not being equal to the care of a second child. Many mothers tell me they want to get pregnant quickly, during the older child's first year, in order to keep from getting too involved with him.

The noted psychoanalyst Erik Erikson once told a mother whose baby I was seeing that he felt no conscientious, caring mother could foresee her ability to split herself in two. She could not anticipate that she would be a good mother to more than one infant at a time, and she would desperately hate to give up an already rewarding relationship with one child for a chancy compromise with two. Thus she naturally would feel both angry and guilty about deserting her first child.

For Mrs. Shaw the pregnancy not only meant a break in an intense and rewarding relationship, but also, since Tom was at a stage where he was becoming more assertive of his independence, she was blaming herself and her "desertion" for all his difficult behavior. Perhaps she could have handled his teasing more easily if she had not been under the physical and emotional strain of the new pregnancy. As it was, her guilty feeling and Tom's negativism combined to make her feel that she had indeed deserted him already.

I tried to clarify some of these matters for Mrs. Shaw, to point out the lack of foundation for what was actually her overreaction. I tried to strengthen her conviction that it would be better for Tom in the long run to have a brother or sister. In addition I could assure her that I foresaw her ability to mother two children and I would help her see her way.

I deliberately did not assure her that her relationship with Tom would be just the same after the baby came. Nor did I assure her that she would be "just as good" a mother, or even the same kind of mother, to the new baby as she had been to Tom. Nor did I say she would love both equally.

And I certainly didn't suggest that Tom needn't feel deserted by her and angry with her and jealous of the new baby.

## *July*

Mrs. Shaw came to the office with Tom, who has a mild ear infection. She is in her sixth month of pregnancy. She is still grieving for her relationship with Tom but seems to be bearing up a little better under his provocations, which are subsiding somewhat.

I asked her how her husband felt about the prospect of a new baby. She said quickly, "You know, I almost think he was jealous of Tom and me and is even a bit glad that we must break it up. He thinks I was spoiling Tom—that diluting my feelings with another child will be better for Tom."

I agreed that it would be better for Tom to have a sibling and share the wealth. I could even reinforce Mr. Shaw's implied hope that he might be more a part of Tom's world after the new baby came. One of the most rewarding things about a second infant for a father is that the older child does turn to him for comfort and fun when much of the mother's time is taken up with the new baby.

As Mrs. Shaw was helping Tom dress after his examination, she asked me, "How can I keep him from being jealous of the new baby?"

I assured her that she *couldn't*—that jealousy was a natural, inevitable state between siblings, and that to assume that one could avoid it was a mistake and a waste of time.

Mrs. Shaw did not reply and I realized that I had been too blunt. I explained that, although one couldn't avoid jealousy, one could help a child as sturdy and solid as Tom to learn to handle it, and I would try to help her do just that. I suggested that she and her husband make an appointment to come in and talk about it.

### August

Mr. and Mrs. Shaw came in and we talked about how to cushion the blow for Tom.

Mrs. Shaw recalled her own jealous feelings about her younger sister, and remembered that she had always hated feeling so angry with her and yet had always resented her mother for bringing her into the house—and here she was doing the same thing to Tom. Her own mother had always tried to stop their fights and to control their jealousy, but had succeeded only in making both of them feel bad for not "loving each other as sisters should."

I pointed out that an older child is not likely to resent the new baby at first. What he resents is the separation from his mother. Even in countries where a mother does not physically leave her home and family to give birth, she does withdraw into herself and in essence leave the family to have her baby and to begin mothering it.

It would help Tom if he could stay in his own home while Mrs. Shaw was in the hospital, rather than being sent to either grandmother's house. We agreed that it would be best if Grandmother arrived a few days before the baby was expected so that she and Tommy could get used to each other's ways. Particularly important would be the fact that Tom's father would be in and out as usual—or, if possible, at home more than usual—and could offer Tom a real anchor. Meanwhile Tom's familiar bed and toys would be symbols of stability for him.

If such an arrangement had not been possible, I would have suggested that Tom be taken in advance for an overnight or weekend visit to the grandmother or relative with whom he would be staying so that he would know his bed and surroundings. And, of course, his father would visit him each day.

Mrs. Shaw had talked to Tom off and on about the baby who would be arriving, and he showed that he had some concept of that. He seemed interested in other people's babies, alternating between showing off for them with silly faces and antics and looking at them hard and seriously and running to bury his head in his mother's lap.

We agreed it was important that Tom be prepared for his mother's impending absence but that there was no reason to talk about it far in advance—a few days before would be ample, given Tom's immature sense of time.

When parents have prepared themselves as well as the older child (or children) for the mother's temporary separation from the family and for the arrival of the new infant, the disruption is bound to be easier for all of them. Parents do not have to feel as guilty and upset and the older child need not lose his or her basic trust in family and environment.

However, this does not amount to a magical avoidance of jealousy and rivalry later on. It is a built-in fact of family life that children compete for the love of their parents. I am sure that most parents, like Mrs. Shaw, have complex feelings left over from their past about their own siblings and wish they could avoid any such rivalry among their own children. Even if they could— and they can't—I'm not sure that they should. In our childrearing we have fostered individuality and intense relationships between parent and child.

Implicit in these two practices is a competitive

approach to self-assertion. In a more communal society these qualities are suppressed, and I am sure that sibling rivalry is less of an issue. But as long as we wish to raise individuals strong and flexible enough to cope with our kind of society, we must accept the inevitability of sibling rivalry. The question is not how to avoid it but whether we can use it as a learning experience for children.

Mrs. Shaw made one more stab at a Utopian world where children love each other unequivocally. If she had become pregnant sooner, when Tom was younger and less aware of her desertion, she asked me, could she have avoided the rivalry?

Many parents ask me that. They want to know the ideal age gap that might prevent competitiveness between children. I always reply that the whole attempt is doomed to failure. Rather, I ask, what age gap will make it easier for you, as parents, to see the two children as individuals who can cope with you and with each other? Can you care for two small babies at the same time, giving each a fair share of yourself? If not, don't have them too close together. Although you feel that number one is too small at a year to realize your desertion, that child will come into his or her own with a blast at a later date, and you will have more than enough rivalry when both are large enough to pound away at each other.

Once in a while a mother of two children who are close together will tell me that there is never any rivalry between them. I always wonder whether there is any deep, positive feeling between them either. Or, I wonder, have the two been treated so similarly that they are lacking in individuality—so that they have nothing to be competitive or jealous about?

## September

Mrs. Shaw gave birth to a fine seven-pound-two-ounce girl. After I checked the baby over, I stopped to see the mother.

Her leave-taking from Tom hadn't been exactly as we had planned it.

She avoided telling Tom until her pains had started, and by then she was so upset that her sad farewell frightened him. He ran away to hide in his room. His mother found him in his crib, clutching his blanket and sucking his thumb, his face turned toward the wall. She was so disturbed that she was unable to talk to him anymore. Then Mr. Shaw went in to Tom, picked him up, hugged him, and said, "Don't worry, Tom. Mother will be gone a few days, but I'll be here. We can play trucks, and I'll read to you at night. And Grandma's staying too."

And then quite spontaneously—he couldn't bear the thought that both of them would be leaving Tom behind—Mr. Shaw said, "Come on, Tom. Hop out and get into the car and let's take Mother to the hospital." Tom brightened. They drove Mrs. Shaw to the hospital and said good-bye to her as she went upstairs with an attendant. Mr. Shaw

took Tom home to Grandma. Then he sped back
to the hospital!

## October

Mrs. Shaw brought Sally in for her shots. The
baby is doing very nicely, Tom, she said, wasn't
doing so nicely—especially during Sally's feeding
times.

When she went home from the hospital Mrs.
Shaw took Tom a new teddy bear. Since she had a
new baby to care for, she thought he might be
encouraged to care for a new cuddly thing too. As
she fed Sally she urged Tom to cuddle his teddy
bear while he sat in the crook of her free arm.
But after a few minutes he became restless and
began to tease his mother. Grandmother tried to
divert him, but he ignored her and instead
became noisier and more demanding. Mrs. Shaw
urged him to play with other toys, with no
success. Tom's initial behavior became a pattern
and Sally's feeding times became a shambles.

Mrs. Shaw told me that, much to her surprise,
she found herself getting angry with Tom and
protective of Sally. After a few such hectic
feedings, she had tried to slip away behind closed
doors. But while Mrs. Shaw was feeding Sally in
another room and Tom could not get to her, he
took to emptying bureau drawers, kitchen
cabinets, and the medicine chest.

I urged Mrs. Shaw to let Tom stay with her
when she was feeding Sally and to try to put up
with his antics, difficult as that might be at first
and "unfair" as it might seem to Sally. If Mrs.

Shaw could go along with his attention-getting efforts, they were likely to disappear, and in any event he obviously needed the attention. I suggested that she be prepared to cuddle him, feed him, talk to him, or read to him during Sally's daytime feedings and use the night feedings to communicate with Sally.

Many mothers say they feel that they are cheating the second baby because they have to lean so far in the direction of the first. But no second baby ever expects as much one-to-one interaction with his mother as the first. Nor, probably, does he or she need it. The first child transmits so much to the baby and surrounds him or her with so much stimulation that it makes up for any diminution in the mother's time or energy.

If Mrs. Shaw could help Tommy get over his initial fury by including him in all her activities with Sally, even giving him a role on her behalf ("Could you please fix the blanket?" . . . "She's fallen asleep—would you wiggle her toes gently and see if she'll wake up?"), he might assume a more protective interest in Sally's development and feel less like the excluded member of a triangle. He might resent Sally a bit less.

Tom's early reaction to Sally was an open bid for equal attention. Many small children put up a better front. They may show nothing or valiantly try to please everyone around them. They handle their feelings by being highly solicitious. When the new infant cries, such an older sibling often will rush to the mother and urge her to feed the baby. The older child will accept chores such as fetching diapers or a bottle or even feeding the infant. These activities are certainly to be encouraged, because the older child feels like a useful part of the new family when he or she undertakes such positive tasks.

To help the older child identify with the grown-ups, the baby can be referred to as "our" baby. One event that can contribute greatly to family solidarity may occur when the new baby begins to respond to the older child. A young mother told me how excited her three-year-old son became when the eight-week-old baby began to choose *him* to smile back at. In fact, infants seem to prefer small children to adults for these early responses. A baby will single out a sibling to watch and gurgle to. Long periods of gurgling and talking to each other help to promote and cement the good side of their relationship.

But let the mother of the "good" older sibling beware! He is certainly much easier to get along with than Tommy. For the time being, family life is peaceful—and that is no mean accomplishment. But let her not fool herself into thinking that she has licked sibling rivalry permanently. As long as the baby stays put where he or she belongs—in the crib—some older siblings will be tolerant and even enjoy collecting kudos for being so nice to their brother or sister. But that doesn't last forever.

### March

At six months Sally is a bubbly, bright and active baby. Mrs. Shaw, who brought Sally in to see me without Tom, had two things on her mind. Trouble A: Tommy a few weeks before, in the midst of a brotherly kiss, bit Sally. Trouble B: Tommy was being impossible to toilet-train.

As I talked with Mrs. Shaw a picture of their current dilemmas emerged.

As soon as Sally reached the "cute" stage—that is, as soon as she began to smile and gurgle at visitors—every adult who came into the house spent his or her time trying to draw this charming response from her. Tom would stand in a corner of the room, watching silently while his erstwhile friends and grandparents made fools of themselves over Sally.

When his father and mother sensed Tom's dismay and loneliness, one or the other would pick him up and give him some concentrated attention. At this point Tom would squiggle to be let down and begin to show off, progressing from silly to noisy and eventually to naughty behavior. As Tommy's carrying-on progressively turned the visitors off, the confusion increased and Mrs. Shaw became embarrassed, then firm, then punitive in an effort to control him. It was during one of these terrible afternoons that Tom had bitten Sally.

After that, Mrs. Shaw said, she never dared leave them alone. But as she redoubled her watchfulness, Tom began to increase his teasing. Most of his affectionate behavior was mixed with aggressive overtones. As Sally began to sit up, he would give her a gentle shove that toppled her. He was very adept at offering her a toy, only to pull it away just as she reached it.

As for the toilet training, it was almost a classic case. Mrs. Shaw had tried to train Tom just before Sally arrived, and he seemed interested and cooperative. When Sally came home Tom refused to go to the toilet again, and was adamant about it for months afterward. After a particularly bad day when Mrs. Shaw got furious with him, he began to whimper in babylike tones, "Change me like you do Sally."

I try to suggest to mothers that there may be ways to dilute the severe reactions and antagonistic feelings of an older child during the first months after the arrival of a new baby.

First, mothers need to be aware that any separation has new overtones. Being sent off to a friend's house or nursery school, which was entirely acceptable before, now becomes exile—an exile in which the child visualizes the pleasure the mother is having with the new baby while he or she is away.

Going to bed at night becomes a heightened separation process, and older children often express their jealous feelings at being put to bed for the sole purpose of letting Mummy and Daddy play with that wretched baby. Waking at night to see what they all are up to is a common reaction. When parents (who, heaven knows, need a break!) go away overnight or for a weekend, or when there is an emergency that takes a mother from the house, the repeated separation appears to be an especially traumatic experience for the older child.

I am not saying that children must be spared

these experiences. Many of them are necessary events in the life of a family. But parents can be aware of their new, heightened implications. When the older child is going back to a play group or to school, the mother should try to free herself to go with him the first time or two— preferably without the new baby, in order to emphasize her wish to be alone with him. At bedtime she and her husband should renew the old rituals of reading and cuddling, letting him regress to being their baby.

When an older child wakens at night, his mother can go to comfort him at first; later she can call to him from her bed, reassuring him that she is there. She needn't allow a nighttime awakening problem to build up, but she does need to acknowledge his extra anxiety. If she has to leave him for medical reasons, Daddy can take him to the hospital to see her through a window or he can talk to her on the phone. The father can spend extra time again reassuring the child that his mother will return—and when she does, the child's increased anxiety about separation must be understood.

A child need not be pushed to achieve new developmental steps such as toilet training. When he is using energy to make a new adjustment, as he surely is with a new baby, he must either stand still or regress in other areas in order to conserve energy for the important adjustment. No small child should be expected to master two steps at once. When a mother can accept his regressive, infantile behavior, she will find that he will play it out for a period, begin to see it as play, and then progress much more quickly to mature behavior. When she refuses to permit the infantile behavior and reacts to it as teasing and competitive, she is likely to prolong the child's need for it.

Special times for him alone with each parent will make up for a great deal of time that must be shared with the baby. Not only can a mother and father spend special periods with the older child, they also can play up the importance of these periods by talking about "the time we will be alone together again." The fact that these times are possible, that you want him and want to be alone with him, may be obvious to the adult, but I can assure you that it isn't obvious to the child. You must let him know it.

Including the infant in the life of the family has many rewards, not only for the older child, for whom it presents more opportunity to get used to the baby, but also for the infant, who will profit from the stimulation of the older child. I need only remind mothers of the marvelous capacity of an infant to shut out what he doesn't want and to take in what he does want in the way of stimuli.

I always suggest that when a mother is busy or out of the room, the baby be placed in an infant seat inside the playpen—not on a table or on the floor—if there is a small brother or sister present. This way the mother has time to get to the baby to save him from assault. Too many "accidents" can happen to a new baby while a mother's head is turned. Such incidents will frighten the older child and heighten his guilty and negative feelings about the baby. Mother should be present when the two are together for any length of time; the older child may tire of pleasing or playing with the baby, and as the negative side of his feelings surge to the fore, he may lash out in some unpremeditated way.

When an older child does hurt the infant, for whatever reason, he needs immediate and understanding consolation. Tommy must have been frightened after biting Sally. He may have hostile, angry feelings about his sister, but they are painful to him. If he is to learn how to handle these feelings and submerge them in favor of his more positive ones, he has to understand the need for and the possibility of controlling them. When his anger suddenly gets out of control, his anxiety frightens him, and without reassurance that this need not happen over and over again, he may well fall into a pattern of acting out his hostile emotions whenever he feels them. This may indeed represent the course of severe sibling rivalry, with all its destructive implications.

## September

Sally was in with a sore throat and slight temperature, cranky and frustrated but still appealing. She is on the verge of walking. Mrs. Shaw says that whenever she teeters by the side of a table and is about to take off, Tom manages to whirl by her, shouting. The combination of noise and rush sends Sally to the ground. She'll walk a little late!

## November

Tom has chicken pox. I made a house call and got a firsthand view of the brother and sister—and Mrs. Shaw—in action.

Sally is obviously at a stage to set Tom's teeth on edge. She is adorable, and no doubt everyone comments on it. And now that she's able to navigate, she gets into everything that Tom has staked out as his own. Like many three-year-olds, Tom is just learning how to share with his peers —but not with his sister.

Tom was building a tower of blocks and had assembled a mass of toys within its ramparts. It was clear that the toys were there to be guarded from Sally. From the other room, writing a prescription, I watched out of the corner of my eye as Sally wobbled toward Tom to join in his play. Tom gathered his toys under him as if they were a nest of precious eggs. As he sat on top of his treasures, he literally growled at the approaching tigress, warning her away. But she came right on, blinded by her adoration for Adonis in his tower. In a moment Tom was kicking her and pummeling her with his fists. She looked surprised and fell onto her back silently, overwhelmed but still half grinning. When Mrs. Shaw rushed in to pick her up, Sally whimpered and clung to her mother. Mrs. Shaw hugged her and called Tom a bad boy.

This demonstration frightened Sally more than Tom's action had. Tom broke down in tears from unspent anger, frustration, chicken pox, and the guilty feelings that his mother's vehemence had produced—heightened, I suspect, by my presence. As Mrs. Shaw saw me to the door, holding her damaged darling, I called good-bye to Tom. He was sitting, alone, on top of his defended tower.

It was perfectly obvious that Sally will soon learn that when she whimpers her mother will appear from several rooms away to rescue her. It is also clear that a pattern can develop here: Sally teases Tom; Tom tortures Sally. Watching the process, one sees that each child may play an equal part as instigator. And one may find that there are rewards for both in the process.

There are many points that can be made about the triangle Mrs. Shaw is setting up when she takes sides with Sally against Tom or Tom against Sally. When she is near enough, the name of the game will be to involve her—the sibling rivalry becomes aimed at the mother. Left alone, most siblings who are old enough to defend themselves will find a way to cope with each other. If a parent is present and ready to interfere, the children's relationship to each other becomes less important than each child's relationship with the mother. Each is more aware of *her* reaction than of each other's. The mother's presence gives them permission to go further than they might without her, for she is there to keep them from going too far. I am convinced that the acute problems of sibling rivalry arise when a mother is too involved in defending each child from the other. Siblings make a better relationship with each other on their own.

Of course, a parent must protect a small child

from injury in a pitched battle. She must stop
fights before feelings build up to such blind
intensity that someone unwittingly is hurt. But in
general, battles are better handled by the
children.

Mrs. Shaw still may ask at this point, "What
will it do to Sally if I leave her to Tom's mercy?" I
would answer that Sally will learn what is safe to
try with Tom and what she must beware of. She
will learn how to defend herself when necessary.
She will even learn how to draw mercy out of
him, and she will be fitted with these wiles for
life.

Mrs. Shaw may also ask, "Is it right for Tom to
manage Sally by the threat of force? Will he think
he can always have everything he wants in that
way?"

You have only to watch (from afar) the kind of
sharing, protectiveness, and care engendered in
an older child who feels responsible for "his" or
"her" baby to realize that Tom would use less, not
more, force with Sally if he were not so sure of
his mother's intervention. He might learn to share
one of his toys with Sally in order to keep her
away from his block tower. He might craftily offer
her three toys in exchange for the one she is
playing with that he wants. He might learn to
comfort her when he has hurt her. All these skills
come more easily when a mother is not hovering
over them, but measuring their interaction before
she jumps in.

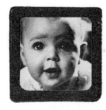 Staying out of
the struggle

Why is the natural competition that occurs
between two children in a family such a difficult
issue for parents in our culture? In the preceding
article, I have tried to point out some of the
reasons that I have sensed and heard from my
discussions with concerned parents. Some of them
bear repeating.

Most parents *who care* a great deal about being
good parents never feel adequate to their children.
They may be able to rationalize to themselves that
they are doing all they can, and all that a child
should need, but basically their caring concern
outweighs their ability to argue it away
intellectually. So, when tension in the household
builds up in the form of sibling rivalry, parents
take it as a sign of their own failure. They feel
that if they had been more adequate parents to
each child, there would be no need for them to be
rivalrous, no need to tease, no need to struggle for
the same toy, no need to come crying with
problems of rivalry. For indeed, the children sense
their parents' vulnerability and *always* attempt to
involve them. As any parent already knows, very
few such fights occur *except* within a parent's
territory. In fact, this very fact points to the
triangular nature of sibling rivalry. *Unless* there
is a target for the struggle, it just isn't worth it to
either child, and each of them can find more

*171*

satisfaction in adjusting to play with the other, *unless* there's a target parent within sight or hearing. This is the rationale for my advice about handling any single episode: simply remove yourself from the scene. Very little rivalry can survive in an empty, targetless environment.

But, if it's as simple as that (and it can be), why can't a loving parent like Mrs. Shaw extract herself? The answer, I hope, is obvious—because she does care and does feel responsible for each of her competing offspring, and when they compete openly for her attention, it strikes at her basic feeling of not having been quite adequate to each of them. In a society like ours where success is at such a premium, where we are all made aware that our children's futures are in our hands in the early years, where guidelines for childrearing are not easy to come by, where everyone is ready to criticize our mistakes as parents but few are prepared to understand our concerns and to help, where even our older children shake us up by pointing to all of our mistakes in rearing them, it is very difficult for a parent to feel confident. So it doesn't surprise me as a pediatrician that the more parents care about the kind of job they are doing, the more vulnerable they are. Any parent who has been through childhood with an older or younger sibling with whom he or she fought and has had the experience of learning how to cope with the constant teasing of someone near in age, remembers the gut reaction of shame and helplessness when the provocateur hits on the right phrase that hurts. And these parents feel

they must protect their own children from ever
going through that "negative" experience. My
question is twofold: *Can* one or *should* one protect
a child from learning how to "cope" with teasing
and rivalry? I don't think children can be
protected and I'm sure they shouldn't be in our
present world. For I feel that learning to compete
and to handle one's own anger and rivalry are a
job that is well-learned in childhood, and is much
more painfully learned as an adult. Perhaps this
fact alone makes it as expensive as it seems to be
to be raised as an only child.

If parents needn't protect their children from
learning about rivalry with each other, but they
can't extract themselves and their own feelings
from a rivalrous situation, what is their role? As I
have indicated, the most difficult *but* most
productive role they can play is that of leaving it
to the children themselves. If they can walk away
from a growing conflict, the children will learn a
lot more than if they stay involved. Parents can
surely attempt to teach the values inherent in
learning to live with each other—such things as
how good it is to be able to depend on each other,
to care for each other when the other is in
trouble, even to learn to love the other (and it is
surely not "natural" to love an intruder). But, if
parents use these adult values as weapons to
attempt to force their relationship in a positive
direction, I can promise nothing but failure. It is
far better to wait until after a rivalrous episode
has resolved itself, and to use any good that
finally results as a way of reinforcing the positive

side. After a fight, when one child is bloody, if and when the other begins to comfort the maimed one, as he or she will if left with him or her, parents often rush in to punish the attacker and to comfort the victim. That surely would be any parent's natural inclination. But by this behavior the parent reinforces the attacker's already overwhelming guilty reaction and forces him or her into a self-protective posture of no longer caring and of blaming the victim. Left alone, this same guilty feeling would have turned to a caring and comforting response toward the victim which could have acted as a learning experience for both of them. The attacker has much more complex feelings at stake than the victim, in any case, and needs to have an opportunity to work them out. With time and with help, he or she can learn an important lesson about dealing with aggression—and its aftermath. When children can learn that by feeling sorry and demonstrating it, you can make up for such an aggressive outburst, they have learned a great deal. An episode that ended with each child in tune with the other could be a more positive step toward sibling attachment than any lesson they would learn from parents.

I realize how difficult it is for parents to stay out of their children's struggles as they veer toward a bloody outcome, but I am convinced not only that fewer and fewer will become bloody, but also that such struggles can have a positive outcome. However, I do not recommend that children be encouraged or even permitted to resort to truly violent rivalry. There are other ways of working out such feelings, and parents can and should point some of them out.

What of the only child—does he or she lose out on an important kind of learning by not having to struggle with siblings? In this era of zero population growth, one or two children spaced widely apart may experience little opportunity for sharing. And they will lose something precious. It is easier to learn to share because you have to, than because you want to. And parents as well do not have to share themselves with single children, so they don't learn some of the necessary lessons of separation, or of leaving the child to work things out for himself or herself. The sense of autonomy and of separation becomes more difficult for such children and for their parents. I would urge parents of single children or of widely spaced ones to be aware of the missed possibilities and to make conscious efforts to provide peers who are aggressive and are matched competition for the single child. I would urge this by the second year and then all along. Learning to share is hardest in the negative, self-protective second year. And this is also a time when two negative self-protective toddlers will learn most from each other and about themselves.

Should one worry when children continue to be openly rivalrous and angry with each other as they grow up? Although I certainly do feel that one never completely outgrows rivalrous feelings about one's siblings, I would be concerned if children continue to be totally unable to get along

as they get beyond six or seven years of age. By
that time, their interests should be spreading out
beyond the home and their peer relationships
should be subsuming more and more of their
interests, and they should be less intensely
involved with such struggles at home. Of course,
there will be fights and struggles off and on, and I
would not look for signs of positive attachment all
the time, but I would expect intervals in which
siblings showed that they had begun to master
some of their rivalry and even their aggression
from time to time. If these signs weren't
beginning to show, a child's use of sibling rivalry
to call attention to himself or herself may well be
seen as a cry for help. Children may be too caught
up in their own problems with anger and with
helpless feelings of not being able to cope with
growing up, with their inability to give up their
own narcissistic concerns in order to make friends
of their own age, and to care for someone beside
themselves. Children who are caught in this stage
of development need extra attention and help
from parents, and from professionals who can
advise their parents. Intense sibling rivalry may
simply be the symptom for such a need.

To summarize, sibling rivalry is not an evil
born of parental failure. It is a fact of family life
as we know it. Parents need to acknowledge its
existence without being frightened or guilty about
it, and then children can learn to do the same. I
would rather advise parents how to use it instead
of pretending that they can "handle" it in a way
that will make it disappear. It can be a major
spur in children's learning to live together,

learning how to share, how to win victories and suffer defeats, how to love and how to cope with their own unloving feelings. It can teach young children what people other than parents are like and how one can live with and care for them. If one hasn't learned this in childhood, it may be far more expensive to learn it as an adult.

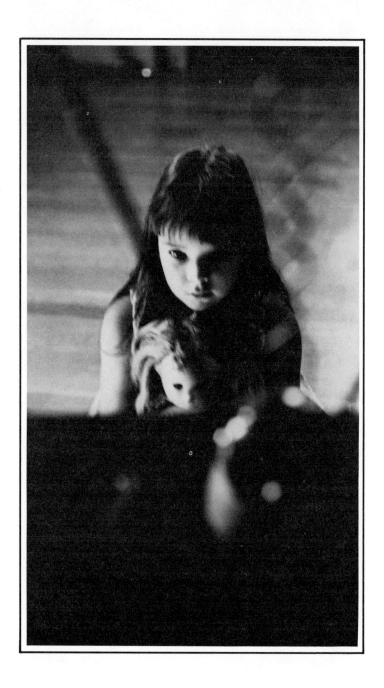

# Chapter 10

# How to tame the TV monster

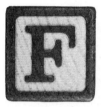or a long time we have known that television plays an important role in the lives of our children. But only within the last few years have we begun to understand how powerful its influence really is, and many of us are worried. Recognizing the problem is one thing; solving it is another.

As a parent and as a pediatrician I think the situation is not hopeless—difficult, yes, but not hopeless. I think there are some positive steps we can take to control this monster medium. Before we get into practical things you can do, however, let me first sketch the basis of my concern about television—about what it is and what it does.

My uneasiness is related to my studies of newborn babies. When they are born, they are thrust from a protective existence inside the mother's womb into a hostile world outside. And given the fact that their major job involves simply trying to achieve some kind of equilibrium between themselves and their new world, it has always amazed me that they are able to interact with the environment in the sophisticated way they do.

From the moment of birth infants are able to take in and process information. They have a set of powerful mechanisms that allow them to control their universe, that allow them to respond with true discrimination to the sights and sounds around. Since they might otherwise be at the mercy of all the stimuli to which they are exposed, they have the capacity to shut out those they judge "inappropriate." (See chap. 5.)

A good example of what I mean by this comes from studies my co-workers and I carried out on newborn infants. We exposed a group of quietly resting babies to a disturbing visual stimulus—a bright operating-room light—placed twenty-four inches from their heads. The light was on for three seconds, then off for one minute, the sequence repeated twenty times; throughout the test the babies were monitored for changes in their heartbeat, respiration, and brain waves. The first time the babies were exposed to the light stimulus, they were visibly startled; however, the intensity of their reaction decreased rapidly after a few times. By the tenth stimulus there were no changes in behavior, heartbeat, or respiration. By the fifteenth stimulus, sleep patterns appeared on the electroencephalogram, although it was clear that their eyes were still taking in the light. After twenty stimuli the babies awoke from their "induced" sleep to scream and thrash about.

Our experiment demonstrated that a newborn certainly is not at the mercy of his or her environment. He or she has a marvelous mechanism, a shutdown device, for dealing with disturbing stimuli: He or she can tune them out and go into a sleeplike state.

But if we can imagine the amount of energy a newborn baby expends in managing this kind of shutdown—energy that could be put to better use —we can see how expensive this mechanism becomes when it is at work all the time.

And if we can realize this, I think, we may be getting to some understanding of the way television works and the way it affects small children. For just like the operating-room light, television creates an environment that assaults and overwhelms children; they can respond to it only by bringing into play their shutdown mechanism and thus they become more passive.

I have observed this in my own children and I have seen it in other people's children. As they sat in front of a set that was blasting away, watching a film with horrors of rapidly varying kinds, the children were completely quiet. Nails bitten, thumbs in mouth, faces pale, bodies tense—they were "hooked." If anyone interrupted, tapped a child on the shoulder to break through the state of rapt attention, he or she almost always would start and might even break down in angry crying. If led away from the set, he or she often dissolved into a combative, screaming, wildly thrashing mass.

Sigmund Freud's daughter Anna, an eminent child analyst, once called such behavior the "disintegration of the ego." Indeed it seemed that whatever ego the child had was being sorely tested at a time like that. And I think the intensity of the reaction is clear evidence of the energy the child is putting into television watching and the shock experienced when his or her attention, locked onto the screen, is broken into.

What bothers me most about television is the passivity it forces on children—the passivity that requires all activity to be produced for them, not by them. And this, I feel, must have a powerful influence on any child's capacity to handle normal aggressive impulses.

By the time a child is five or six years old, his or her fantasies are already as violent as those in any horror movie adults might construct, and his or her sexual fantasies can match anything presented in a grade-C movie. The violence and adult forms of sexuality displayed on television mobilize these fantasies together with all the fear and anxiety that go with them.

I feel this is one of the grave dangers of all the violence and sexual activity to which children are exposed—not that children are taught anything new by it, but that it strikes at very primitive impulses and mobilizes them, and leaves children with no way to give healthy expression to them. It comes down to the fact that television gives children two choices—they can actively suppress their feelings or they can ineffectually play them out.

No wonder, then, that a child comes away from a set believing that physical violence is a perfectly acceptable form of self-expression.

When we adults watch a television program—or a movie, for that matter—we do not always respond to what we see at the very moment it is being presented. Particularly if the material is disturbing or otherwise provocative, we often avoid immediate confrontation with it. But at a later time—an hour or so afterward, perhaps even the next day—we think about what we have seen. We reflect on it and compare it with our own experiences and our own store of ideas. We make sense of it first and then decide whether it is true for us.

But children can't bring this sort of control to what they see on television because their intellectual development hasn't taken them that far. They can't delay their response until they have mulled it over and tested it in their mind; they can't go back to it later. They are hooked into the experience of the moment; they give themselves totally to what they are viewing. The sights and sounds coming from the television screen wash over them then and there, and they can't protect themselves, as we can, with intellectual detachment. They are forced to be passive receivers.

In this sense, watching television for children is totally different from reading—which might seem to be a similar passive activity. But there are a number of very important differences. First of all, when young children are reading, they are putting into operation newly acquired skills, and this in itself requires active participation. As they struggle over each syllable, each word, they try to relate it to other syllables and words, to other ideas, they have learned. Though physically undemanding, reading requires children to be mentally alert, to think, to bring to it something of themselves.

And then, of course, the material presented in children's books is totally different from the kind that fills the television screen. Usually there is nothing so threatening, nothing so overwhelming, nothing that is so likely to stir up a child's unconscious fantasies. The authors and editors of children's literature are very scrupulous about this today. They are concerned about issues in child development; they are concerned about the age appropriateness of the material they publish, and often indicate that a book is recommended for children in a certain age bracket.

But this is not true for television, which for the most part does not take into account differences in age and in sensitivity among its young viewers. Adventure movies, even cartoons, may contain a level of violence and brutality that may not faze a seven- or eight-year-old, because at that age children can make a clearer distinction between what is real and true to life and what is not. But for a three- or four-year-old, such distinctions are not possible. Younger children may watch a cartoon show and come away disturbed and upset, though an adult—or an older child, for that matter—would consider it totally harmless. They cannot understand why Tom keeps hitting Jerry; they worry about how much it hurts. As a result they themselves feel confused and vulnerable.

Still, even though we have to face the fact that television is not the best medium for a child to be exposed to, it does have an undeniable importance in the world today. From all the evidence it looks as if it's going to be around for a very long time, and we'll simply have to come to terms with it. But this does *not* mean that we as parents must throw up our hands in dismay and resignation. There are a few outstanding television programs for children, which means that "quality" is possible—if we demand it. Further, we *can* take some steps now to control what and how much television our children watch.

So now let's talk about what's right with television. The first time I was exposed to such programs as "Sesame Street," "Mister Rogers' Neighborhood," and, more recently, "The Electric Company," and "Zoom," I began to be aware of the real potential for good that television programs can provide. Instead of being overwhelming, depleting, passive experiences, these programs demonstrated that small children could have warming times and learn exciting things—about their world and about themselves— in a period of television watching.

I first became aware of Mister Rogers when one of my four-year-old patients quoted him during his entire examination in my office. He was a boy who had been frightened of me on previous visits but was trying hard to master his anxiety this time. After I applied the cold stethoscope to his chest he nodded and said, "Just like Mister Rogers." When I used the earpiece, he winced but allowed it, saying, "Just like Mister Rogers." Before his shot he said, "Mister Rogers said it was okay for kids my age to cry for a shot. Do you think it is, Dr. Brazelton?"

Not to be outdone by this mythical Mister Rogers, I said, "Of course it is, Dan. And you know what? If you look the other way and let out a yell when I do it, it won't even hurt too much." These maneuvers worked to distract him. He yelled for a minute after the shot, then stopped and with a straight face said, "You're almost as good for kids as Mister Rogers."

By this time I wanted very much to congratulate a man who could prepare a child for a frightening experience by using a television program. By demonstrating what might happen on a visit to the doctor and by giving suggestions about how to face up to the anxiety and the pain it might bring, he had helped this boy through an ordeal and given him a chance to be proud of himself.

"Sesame Street" was literally shoved down my throat day after day by one three-year-old after another who read the letters from my eye chart with the musical phrase appropriate to each letter. I have watched "Sesame Street" myself, and I can see what a powerful teaching medium it is.

I do not feel that all the programs children watch must be "learning" experiences. Children really need to relax after a day in school; they must have some "throwaway" time. And I think they would find it in other ways—in comic books, for example—even if we could construct enough educational programs to fill the prime-time hours.

But it does seem that children really might prefer to be offered "good" and thoughtful programs for their selection. This is pointed up by the enormous number who watch repeats of "Sesame Street" or of "Mister Rogers' Neighborhood," who will cut off a war drama or a stirring love story their parents are watching to tune in to these repeats. My children say, "But, Dad, these programs are for *me.*"

I feel that all you parents should try to acquaint yourselves with the programs that are being offered in your area, and then you can play an active part in your child's television viewing. Every Sunday or Monday, for example, you and your child could sit down with a guide to the week's shows and discuss them together. For each day select one or two programs that you both agree would be entertaining and worthwhile. If your child insists on something you don't think is suitable, gently but firmly discuss your reasons.

You could also make your selections on a daily basis, gearing your choices around the day's events and your child's mood. For a quiet day he might need a soothing storyteller or a visit with Mister Rogers. For a learning day, "Sesame Street" or "The Electric Company" might be more appropriate. But whichever method you decide to use, after the program follow up with a discussion about what went on and an assessment of its quality. In this way you can make the experience a deeper and more meaningful one for your child.

Ideally, of course, it would be best if you could actually be there with your child and watch the program along with him or her, because your presence and obvious concern will give a deeper and more human dimension to what is essentially an isolating experience. Perhaps you could see to it that you are in on at least one or two full programs per week. I realize, though, that it is not always possible for a busy parent to do this, so I would urge you then at least to try to be available during these times. Let your child know in advance that if he wants you for any reason— because he is disturbed by something he is watching, because he wants something explained, because he just needs you there with him—you'll certainly come. When and if this does happen, do sit down and *listen* to him, trying to understand the concerns of his that have been stirred up.

Perhaps you might also think about the ways in which you can use television as a positive and cementing force within your family. For example, most mothers need a baby-sitter at certain times of the day. They need the relief from demands of housekeeping and childrearing, the time to prepare the evening meal, an organizing force to bring children down from the exciting experiences of the day to a more relaxed, comfortable state. Appropriate programs could help do this *and* provide children with a worthwhile experience. Programs that bring all the members of the household together after

supper can be an opportunity for valuable
interaction—for example, word games or guessing
games in which all ages can participate actively
*as a family.*

There is just one more point I would like to
make. I believe one hour a day is the maximum
amount of time children up to the age of five or
six can spend in front of a television set before
they begin to show the signs of depletion and
exhaustion I mentioned earlier. But parents, in
particular mothers, must always be on the lookout
for the symptoms. Whenever they appear, you can
be certain that your child has had too much, and
you must reduce the television-watching time
accordingly.

In attempting to outline some of the problems
television causes and in trying to give some ways
of coping with them, I am not suggesting that we
eliminate television altogether—I certainly am not
that much of an ostrich. But I would urge all of us
who are parents to take a more active role in this
part of our children's lives. We must replace the
almost total lack of control that exists today with
individual choice, with the freedom to decide
upon or refuse a program. This kind of active
participation on the part of the parent, as well as
the child, may begin to make television the
valuable experience it should be.

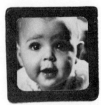 # The parents'
# responsibility

Since the preceding article was written, the
grass-roots organization Action for Children's
Television, made up of concerned parents, has
pressed the Federal Communications Commission
to set limits on programs for children. The
number and duration of commercials in
prime-time programs have been limited, and the
content of the commercials is more carefully
regulated. I was intrigued and delighted by the
report of Harvard Business School researcher,
Scott Ward, who reported that children by the
ages of four to six years had already learned that
commercials were to be attended to differently
and were not necessarily to be believed. Perhaps
in our complex society there is value in learning
early that the adult world around you is full of
double-talk and complicity, but it seems a painful
lesson, nonetheless, at such an early age.

There is a ground swell to restrict the kind of
programming for children's prime time—to
eliminate much of the raw violence and sexual
acting-out which furnishes the excitement in most
of the programming in the United States. To
change this is a more difficult task, but I would
not put anything past the efforts of a group of
aroused, concerned parents. And the effective
pressures which Action for Children's Television
has been able to muster have been another
reminder to me of the strengths inherent in the

democratic process when it is at its best. There
are efforts now at the government level to back
programs aimed at education for young parents,
and we may soon begin to see more and more
programs about childrearing which will have
content that is rewarding enough to hold their
own in the competitive television field. With the
advent of cable television and home sets for
cassettes which will allow a wider choice of
programs, parents and children may have a richer
field from which to choose.

What will this kind of choice mean to children?
Certainly it will provide them with an opportunity
to make more individual choices. And the very act
of choosing makes the involvement more active.
Since the cassettes must be provided by parents
and choices of cable programs must be made
from a wide range, there is also considerable
opportunity for parental involvement. Not just in
the area of supervision or limitations, but in the
areas of mutual choice and involvement. Parents
and children will have the chance to work
together and find programs for the entire family.
Since television is here to stay, and much of a
family's recreational time is going to be spent
with the television set, perhaps our best use of
television in the future may be to cement the
family. In the past in our own family as in many
others, television produced a strong splitting
effect. I deplored the prevalent programs as well
as the powerful seductive attraction they hold for
children. And I reacted by trying to limit their
watching time (which I do still believe in doing)
and by scoffing at their choices of programs. But

more recently, as I began to relax and participate
with them, the programs chosen have often been
ones which we all like, rather than the violent
massacres watched earlier. We have had fun
together and even discussions following some
complex point in "Upstairs, Downstairs," or an old
movie from "our day." If, indeed, the caliber of
children's programs can be upgraded and more
choice provided, the opportunity for planning
television time for the whole family offers a real
challenge. I would urge parents not to fall into the
most obvious trap—that of setting up nothing but
educational, learning programs. For any child
worth his salt would see through that and would
rapidly lose interest rather than capitulate. If the
choices were made "by committee," by consensus
of all of the family, they could become a focus for
family participation. And this is a bonus for any
family.

The problem of commercialism and the impact
of exaggerated advertising claims should also be
faced by all responsible parents. Dr. Richard
Feinbloom, Medical Director of the Family Health
Care Program of Harvard Medical School, wrote a
letter, submitted by Action for Children's
Television to the Federal Trade Commission for
its hearing on the "Impact of Advertising on
Consumers" in November 1971, expressing his
concern that all advertising directed to young
children is "misleading" because children
normally distort reality in accordance with their
own immature view of the world:

To children, normally impulsive, advertisements for appealing things demand immediate gratification. An advertisement to a child has the quality of an order, not a suggestion. The child lacks the ability to set priorities, to determine relative importance, and to reject some directives as inappropriate. It is no wonder that children are unable to make a mental correction for the distortion of a piece of merchandise as presented on television, particularly when it is dramatically portrayed with booming voices of announcers, excited child participants and rousing musical background.

A medium which could be a powerful educational tool to inform the American public of good health and nutrition is instead a vehicle for falsehood, misinformation and misleading persuasion. Television advertising presents several dangers to the health of children—the most significant are dental caries, the exclusion of more nutritious foods from the diet, obesity, and other health problems which arise in adulthood as a result of a taste for sweets acquired during childhood.

Preschool children are just too young to comprehend the intricacies of commercialism on their own programs and too inexperienced to make reasoned consumer judgments, no matter how much information they are given.

*The Family Guide to Children's Television,* written by Evelyn Kaye and Action For Children's Television (New York: Pantheon Books, 1974),

contains excellent advice for parents on how to
deal with commercials:

> Watch commercials with children and try to put the
> exaggerated claims into perspective. "You know
> that film is speeded up and no car can really go
> that fast." Or, "Isn't that the toy in the cereal that
> broke the last time we got it?"
>
> Teach children to write their own commercials and
> reason out why certain kinds of statements are
> made.
>
> Analyze the specific appeal of the commercial. "I
> bet everyone thinks they'll get all those friends if
> they buy that game, but of course they don't." Or,
> "How can any food make you grow big so fast—
> that's ridiculous."
>
> Take children to the store and compare the ad with
> the actual product, if you think this will be
> effective. Some parents feel that this is too tempting
> and that they will end up buying the product
> because of pleading from the child, even if they feel
> it has been misrepresented.
>
> Only watch noncommercial children's television so
> that young children won't be exposed to
> commercials.

The most important message from the research
and thoughtful assessment that this parent group
has done is (1) that television for children is a
powerful force that is here to stay, and (2) that we
as parents must feel as a major responsibility the
job of teaching our children how to assess and
incorporate the good from the bad. To do this,

they need our efforts in a cooperative learning venture with them. We cannot protect them from television but we can help them learn about it for themselves.

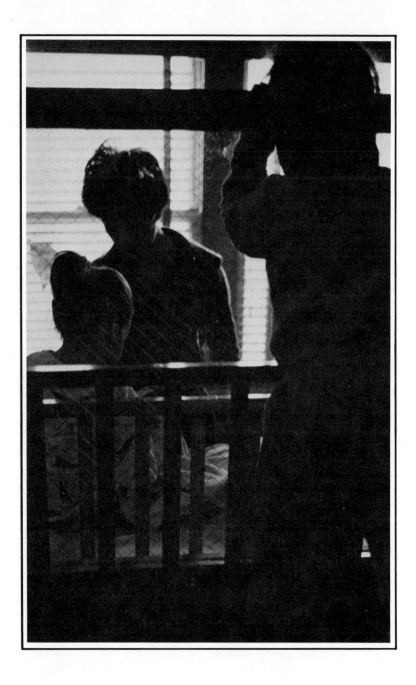

# Chapter 11

# If your child goes to the hospital

ommy has to have his tonsils and adenoids out next week. He's scared and I'm scared. How do I prepare him—or should I? Should I try to stay on the ward with him? I'm so upset, I want to cry when I even think about it!"

Mrs. Landis was an earnest, capable young mother who wanted to do the best she could for her children. Five-year-old Tom had had so many earaches and prolonged sieges from infected tonsils and adenoids that we all were desperate. He had spent the winter on antibiotics. And now he could no longer breathe through his nose because of the enlarged adenoids; his snoring at night rocked the household. He could barely hear when he was spoken to. As he sat quietly in my office, he was washed-out-looking, exhausted—a pitiful version of the vigorous child he had been last year.

Despite our attempts to avoid an operation, nothing else would do but to remove the huge adenoids obstructing his breathing and blocking the internal ducts to his ears. All of us were ready to do anything to prevent a repetition of the winter we'd just been through, even Tommy. He looked forward to the time when he would feel well again, and seemed to understand that there was no alternative. His quiet passivity was like the patience of a much older person who is resigned to doing anything for some kind of relief —*any* kind.

Mrs. Landis, an intelligent, caring mother, was well aware of the potentially damaging effects on a developing child's emotional life that hospitalization can have, with its separation from home and parents and attendant pain and illness. And certainly I agree. At the same time I have strong feelings that a child can learn some pretty positive things from an experience in the hospital and from an operation if they are handled in the right manner.

A great deal of what children learn about themselves comes in stressful situations. And if a hospitalization teaches them that they can cope with pain and being in a strange, frightening place away from home, that they can manage for themselves at times, that doctors and nurses want to help even though they hurt them, it can help them gather confidence in themselves and in other people and it will be a positive experience in learning how to master their world.

But it's important that the adults in the children's environment help them as much as

they can. The questions Mrs. Landis asked me
showed that she was trying to do this. She was
preparing herself, as well as Tom, for the
impending hospitalization, and implicit in what
she asked was a belief that if she did the right
things, she could soften the blow for Tommy. I
heartily agreed, and I could answer her first
question without any qualms. She certainly must
prepare Tommy for his hospital stay with as
much information as she had.

In most pediatrics hospitals there are booklets
for parents that give details about procedures that
can be expected. I have even wished that we
could set up preadmission visits to hospitals for
children who were going to be operated on.
Actually seeing what might be a frightening bit of
equipment ahead of time, particularly in the
company of one's parents, can be very reassuring.

We know, for example, that children who
undergo cardiac surgery do much better in the
critical postoperative period if they have been
shown an oxygen tent beforehand and allowed to
get into it, if they have been taken into the
recovery room and the room where they will
receive treatment *and* if they are introduced to a
child who has been through it all and is
recovering. This last step is of great importance,
for children are like adults in that they can
overcome a great deal of anxiety and pain if they
can identify with someone who has experienced
them.

The Boston Children's Museum has a very
popular exhibit that gives children the
opportunity to play at being sick in a hospital

room. It consists of very little besides a hospital bed, a collection of white coats and a few stethoscopes, but it is always crowded, and at any one time you can hear a child who's been in a hospital proudly telling his awestruck companions about his experiences. I am sure that, superficial as it is, this exhibit becomes a tremendously reassuring memory for a frightened child when he suddenly must be admitted in pain to a hospital bed.

Mrs. Landis winced as I suggested that she warn Tom about the needles and the injections he would receive, about her having to leave him at the time of operation, about the sore throat he would have after it was over. "But wouldn't it just scare him to tell him in advance? And wouldn't it be easier for me to comfort him after it was over and to help him *then?*"

I said it wasn't necessary to tell Tom more than a day or so in advance, but it was important for him to be told. For a child the unknown and unexpected is far more frightening than even the painful ordeal of surgery and hospitalization for which he is prepared. In addition to the anxiety dispelled by preparation for each step in such an experience, the child's trust in his parents and in their ability to protect him is reinforced tremendously by seeing that they are not overwhelmed by this strange, frightening experience.

When we sampled a group of parents who were scheduled to bring their small children to the Boston Children's Hospital Medical Center for admission and who had been urged to prepare

these children with a booklet explaining the
hospital and its procedures, we found that only 15
percent had done so. We tried to find out why
these well-intentioned parents had not acted on
our suggestion. In each case they shyly admitted
that they themselves couldn't face the impending
separation and trauma, and therefore couldn't
face up to a discussion of it with the child. We
knew it was important to the child that his or her
own mother or father prepare him or her, and
finally we arranged to be with these parents while
they read the booklet to their child—often with
tears in their eyes.

The value to each of the children after they
were on the ward was so obvious to us that we
have continued to press parents to prepare their
children in this way. With such preparation
children do not become as frightened or as
withdrawn; they eat, sleep, and recover better
from their illnesses, both in the hospital and after
they return home.

I remember one little boy who sat bolt upright,
rocking in his crib after an operation, sucking his
thumb and clinging to a scarf that his mother had
left with him. As he rocked and whimpered in
pain, he kept singing a song over and over to
himself. When I leaned down to listen, I could
hear the whispered words: "My mama told me
this would happen." The fact that his mother had
prepared him in advance for some of the things
he could expect helped soothe him. He seemed to
cling to her words and to the piece of her clothing
as if she were there.

In short, I urged Mrs. Landis to find out as

many details as she could about the things
Tommy would have to do, where he would stay,
how long he would be there, what kinds of
medication and anesthetic he would have. She
agreed to explain to him on the day before he was
to be admitted all that she had learned. If he
asked questions, which we hoped he would, she
was to answer him as truthfully and completely
as she could. I urged her to call me if she
floundered or felt like wavering, so that I could
remind her of how important all this was to
Tommy.

"Is there anything else I can do to make it
easier for Tom?" she then asked me. I knew that
when Tom came in for checkups he always had
with him a beloved teddy bear that was worn and
frayed and losing its stuffing. I urged her to wash
his toy and to sew up the edges so that it would
not lose its contents all over his hospital bed. I
wanted it to be respected by the hospital
personnel as an important companion for Tommy
in distress. A child's own precious things, own
clothes, and even a picture of the family can be of
great comfort at such a time.

In answer to her question about whether she
should be with him in the hospital, I was very
definite. "Of course you should. This is a time
when a child needs security and comfort more
than any other. Why should he not have it from
you and his father?"

Mrs. Landis replied that the hospital where
Tommy was going really didn't want parents
around. The hospital personnel had said that the
nurses and doctors knew the most about caring

for a sick child and that parents often interfered by being too fluttery and anxious, passing on their own anxiety to the child. She also had been told that children cried more when parents were with them, that they were quieter and could rest and recover better without them. Because Tom was to be in the hospital only two days, the staff had advised strongly that it was better for him to be left alone to recover and to be gathered up the day after the operation.

When I asked Mrs. Landis what she thought about all this, she said, "Well, I was ready to buy their explanations. I kept thinking that it *is* my fault Tommy has been sick so much. He really may do better with the more competent medical staff, because I certainly wouldn't know how to care for him. And I'm sure he would cry more if I was there. But after talking to you, I realize I shouldn't be afraid to fight to stay with Tom."

In her rather sad acceptance of the hospital's dicta I could see the emotional torment caring mothers and fathers suffer when their child is sick—the feeling that somehow they are responsible for what has happened, the sense of helplessness and inadequacy, the guilt.

Of course parents are frightened and feel inadequate and helpless when their child is sick, but I do not believe they will pass on their anxiety to the child if the hospital staff helps to relieve it. Parents tend to overreact, to become combative and belligerent, only when doctors and nurses do not attempt to understand what they are going through. Then they do indeed become problems on the ward and can interfere with the optimal care of their child. But in hospitals where the staff is trained to understand these natural, healthy feelings in distraught parents and where there is provision for incorporating the parents into the care of the sick child, these same "helpless" parents can be a major asset.

In the past few years children's hospitals have begun to change drastically—to include parents on the wards, to plan more active programs for children, which attempt to alleviate the potential psychological effect of illness and separation from home. Organizations of parents, such as Parents Concerned for Hospitalized Children, and Children in Hospitals, have formed to press for changes in hospital procedures—to treat the total child rather than just the disease.

In the Parent Care Unit of Riley Hospital for Children, in Indianapolis, Indiana, mothers and fathers learned to care for their sick child while all of them are under the safe supervision of a knowledgeable staff. There's obvious value to ill children not only in having parents nearby, but also in having them in the familiar role of taking care of them. They even may be able to see themselves in their old healthy image rather than in the new, sick one. And there is obvious value to the hospital—not only have costs of hospital care at Riley been cut in half as a result of parents' participation, but children improve more quickly.

I do *not* feel that children do better with a stranger, no matter how competent, even though they may indeed cry less with someone they don't know than with their parents. For one thing, I am sure it is not harmful for children who are miserable or in pain to cry. In fact I happen to think crying is good for them at such a time. It stirs up their vascular and respiratory systems to a vigorous response that may even speed recovery. But it also gives them a feeling of being able to do something about their misery, of being able to protest. When they do receive comfort and do begin to recover, they may feel it is partly *because* they protested. Protest is a healthy mechanism!

As long as children are protesting, fighting for their rights, crying when it is safe to do so, I am content that they are putting up the healthiest battle they can to come out of such an event without too much psychological scarring.

And on the basis of Mrs. Landis' report, I cannot agree with the hospital policy that two days is too short to worry about. For a child any separation, particularly under frightening and painful conditions, is too long to ignore. Most hospitals are aware of the need to change such outdated practices as keeping parents away, and they will adjust if a parent stands firm.

I urged Mrs. Landis to demand that she be allowed to stay with Tommy. She wouldn't have to press for a bed or a rooming-in arrangement—she could prop herself up in a chair for the night or trade off half the night with her husband. As Tom became accustomed to his new surroundings, after the first night he might not even need one of his parents with him. But I wanted *her* to demand the option and not leave it up to the already biased hospital personnel.

I warned Mrs. Landis that even if she were allowed to stay on the ward, the staff might continue to be unaccepting of her and that she mustn't expect them to allow her to do things for her child. But even if she were stripped of her role as mother to Tommy, her very presence as an anchoring reassurance would be of vital importance to him. If she could prove to the doctors and nurses that her presence was comforting to him and that she needn't get in the way of their doing a good job for him, perhaps she might affect their future policy for other parents.

Certainly there are many situations in which it isn't possible for a parent to stay with a child— such as when a mother has other small children at home and no one to leave them with; or when a child must be hospitalized for a long, stressful period and a parent's constant presence could drain the rest of the family of resources, both financial and psychological.

In these cases there are other ways of helping the hospitalized child. Friends or relatives, especially grandmothers, can substitute for the mother. On the children's wards of some hospitals there is a program for "foster grandparents" funded by ACTION, the Federal agency for volunteer programs, from which both generations profit; and in others there are "play ladies," who make a special effort to involve the child in therapeutic play around the issues of the illness and separation from family. But the emphasis of the entire team concerned with the child's recovery must be on the psychological as well as physical recovery.

The age of the child who must be hospitalized

may influence the kind of concerns he or she has.
For children under five or six separation from
home and parents is an even more terrifying
aspect of the experience than the pain or illness
they must endure, and from four years on, fears of
being damaged or hurt begin to be of more and
more importance.

For five-year-old Tommy the concerns about
separation and about mutilation are both
operating. Having his mother or father nearby
will help decrease his anxiety about separation,
and at the same time may give him the feeling
that he has some protection against the danger of
being mutilated. To help him further, his parents
must try to make him understand the difference
between his fears about losing a necessary part of
himself and the reality of losing a useless and
unnecessary part of himself.

As our talk came to an end, Mrs. Landis asked,
"What can I expect from Tommy when he comes
home from the hospital—will he be angry with
me and hard to cope with?" This question was
harder to answer than the others. Indeed, Tommy
may be angry with his mother when he comes
home, and he might reward her efforts to comfort
and reassure him with negative and angry
behavior. As Mrs. Landis had showed me her
concern about his turning on her, I was afraid
she'd be upset when he did. So I tried to help her
understand that he had no other way to work out
his anxiety or his pent-up anger.

Children rarely blow up in the hospital,
although they may fight and protest valiantly. It
isn't until they return home and are safe that they

dare to begin to show their real feelings, and they nearly always take them out on the safest people around—their parents. This is a healthy mechanism, and it may help Mrs. Landis to know that it is. Still, it is hard to take a child's furious temper tantrums as a reward for having struggled to help him or her make it through such an ordeal.

It is likely that the behaviors Tommy will show will be subsumed under a mechanism called "regression." He may begin to act like a baby—he may cry a lot and cling to either or both parents; he may become more violent and unrestrained in his treatment of his younger brother; he may begin to wet his bed again or to suck his thumb; he may want to be carried or rocked as he did when he was much younger. These regressive behaviors serve a real purpose for Tom. By returning to an earlier level of adjustment, he can conserve his own energy and gain more attention from those around him in order to recover from the demands of the hospital experience.

Parents must see these behaviors for what they are. Mrs. Landis will need to put up with them for a while, to help Tommy understand why he needs them and then to encourage and support him to want to grow up again. Punishment for them might well get rid of them, but only by shoving them underground, where they will not serve the purpose for which he needs them—to help him recover his threatened image of himself.

In a study of normal children, over 50 percent were found to use regressive behavior during the entire six-month recovery period after a hospitalization, no matter how brief it was. This means that it is a pretty normal and healthy way for children to stand still while they gather energy to move forward again.

I urged Mrs. Landis to continue to talk to Tommy about his experiences after he came home, to urge him to play them out, worry them out if it was necessary. Primarily, I felt it important that she and Tom's father be aware that this might well be a scary experience no matter how well they prepared and supported him. But if *he* could see it as one he had got through, had conquered, had been able to rely on them to help him conquer, *then* he could remember it as a real learning experience—a learning how to cope with his own world, no matter what it dealt him!

Parents who wish further information on how to improve conditions for children in hospitals can write to The Association for Child Care in Hospitals (P.O. Box 347 Cleveland, Ohio, 44127) which is made up of doctors, nurses, hospital administrators, and so forth, all working to improve the experience of hospitalization for children. A lay group, called Children in Hospitals (31 Wilshire Park, Needham, Mass. 02192) has organized to assist parents in coping with hospitalization problems.

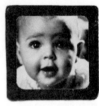

# Guidelines
# for parents

Twenty-five years ago, Drs. Robertson and Bowlby
in England and Dr. D. G. Prugh in Boston began
to fight for parents to stay with their children in
hospitals. They saw needless reactions to
separation in hospitalized children as interfering
with their recovery from illness and prolonging
the recovery period at home. They were at the
forefront of a struggle to counteract medical
practices that had isolated children from parents
half a century before. Nursing and medical care
were not able to provide the important caring
environment that made for recovery from illness.
There have been real strides in hospital care for
children as we have become aware of the
importance of supporting a child's reaction to
illness, to separation, and to the fears of
mutilation that occur around a hospitalization.

In the past few years, studies have shown that
at least 25 percent of hospitalized children can
actually profit psychologically from
hospitalization—if it is handled properly. Such
positive benefits come about from increased
self-confidence in the child from having mastered
the anxiety of hospitalization and illness, as well
as from the correction of defects or conditions for
which he or she is hospitalized. This indication
that children can actually gain from a traumatic
experience makes me want to press toward

environments for sick children that can support this sense of mastery.

We are certain now that the scars of illness and hospitalization can be far-reaching in children's emotional development. Some of the symptoms that are the sequel to an illness or a hospitalization come under the heading of regression: bed-wetting, soiling, night waking, retreat from recently learned developmental steps, such as walking or talking. In fact, I always warn parents that they can expect small children to give up the most recent steps they have accomplished and that they will have to relearn them all over again, after they have recovered from the regressive psychological effects of their illness. Other symptoms result from the anxiety of being ill and hospitalized. They come out as tics, increased thumb sucking, masturbation, head banging, or as night terrors or daytime fears. Even more severe symptoms may be symptoms of apathy, increased sleeping, and passivity. I prefer to see children who have been ill and hospitalized come home fighting. If they can work out their fears and anxiety by some kind of protest, I am sure that they will suffer less in the long run. The reactions of regression, of apathy and withdrawal may not even show up at the time of an illness, but may come out after the child is safely at home again.

We must assume that all children are vulnerable to the anxiety of being ill and damaged, of being separated and even of being discarded. All children unconsciously feel that an illness is retribution for having been "bad." (Just as parents feel that it is their fault.) In developing societies an illness is taken as the result of bewitchment or of the evil eye inflicted by one's neighbor. If one pursues this, it is easy to see that this is a way of blaming your neighbor for your own guilty feelings at being ill or damaged. In the same way, children blame themselves for being sick and hospitalized. When self-depreciation is intolerable, they blame their parents. But this very blaming becomes frightening in itself. For if a parent is indeed responsible, it may be some sort of confirmation of a child's most fundamental fear—that he isn't wanted, and is rejected because he's bad or no good. When parents allow themselves to be caught in hospital policy that excludes them from being with their sick child, this is a powerful confirmation of such fears.

Bowlby points to three stages of hospitalization in children. The first is that of protest in which the child fights hard about everything that is happening to him—he or she cries, struggles, refuses to give in to the routines of hospitalization. The second is that of apathy and compliance. One often sees children in hospitals who are too good, who dare not protest any longer, and who try to please everyone around them. The last and most serious stage is that of withdrawal and of giving up. That each of these reactions has its problems and may even hinder the child's recovery probably doesn't need to be questioned. However, children who protest are likely to be exciting physiological responses that will aid their bodies in fighting infection or bring about more rapid healing. But withdrawn, apathetic children frighten me when I realize how slowed down all of their bodies' responses to recovery must be.

Hospital personnel may hide behind the excuse that parents' presence brings out more protesting behavior, and that this behavior interferes with their routine and the child's recovery. Parents should not accept this excuse. If their presence interferes with the hospital routine, perhaps that routine needs to be reevaluated. And, as a physician, I am sure that protest is healthier for recovery than are the alternative apathetic responses. When a child's protest is too difficult for the hospital and hinders therapy, one can find other outlets for it. For instance, a burned child who must have painful dressings changed, can unnerve the hospital team with too much agonized screaming. A parent's role may then become that of preparing the child to try to master his or her agony at the time, and to express protest later in other ways—such as talking about it, playing it out in aggressive games, and so forth. But even if these fail, I would rather see a child still fighting than one who has become quietly resigned and "too good." And the best insurance against this is having a member of the family there who can support, encourage, and explain each step of the way.

What if a parent cannot be on hand for a child's hospitalization—what then? For many parents, being away from home and other small children becomes such a hardship that the price seems almost too great. In these cases, I would still urge that some arrangement be made so that you can be on hand for a small part of the child's day. Then, prepare the sick child for your coming as precisely as you can, tell him or her why you can't be there more of the day, and *be sure* you do arrive at the predicted time. When you must leave, explain it ahead of time, and make clear when you are going and when you will be back. It may be easier for you not to hear the child's protest at your leaving, to slip away or to lie about your going, but this doesn't make up for the child's feeling of disappointment and desertion.

Since many hospitals still fight a parent's demand that he or she be hospitalized with the child, to be present may become a struggle with hospital personnel. One of the subtler ways that hospitals reject parents even while they are openly accepting them is to make them feel as if they were in the way, and were interfering with the child's good care. Parents who are determined to support their children end up by feeling they may be doing more harm than good. A mother who is tense about her child's illness may be in no mood to accept this, and she may want to fight about it. Friction begins to build up around the child which may indeed be detrimental. I feel it may help parents to understand why nurses and doctors may unconsciously resent their presence. To understand this feeling of resentment, you must remind yourself that any good pediatric nurse or physician will have competitive feelings with you as the child's parent. Each adult who cares about a child will feel he or she can do better by that child than any other adult. This is at the base of caring. And so a caregiver may resent other caregivers and try to shove them out. If a mother wants to preserve the caring relationship for the child which the staff may feel, she may have to accept some of their unconscious resentment. It takes a sense of humor and of understanding to be able to put up with this at a time when your own anxiety needs understanding from the hospital staff.

When the spirit of a pediatric unit makes parents feel welcome, they don't mind discomfort nearly as much. Rollaway beds or chairs in which to spend the night, poor toilet facilities, little privacy can all fade. Occasionally a parent falls apart and becomes a real deficit—both to the ward and to her child. But then other parents can step in and help her. And, if the pediatric unit is set up for it, individual or group support can be available to such a parent. An ideal ward would have a trained worker available to conduct group discussions for all parents of sick children so that they can understand the universal dynamics of taking care of an ill, frightened, and demanding child.

The ideal pattern would be for mothers or fathers of small children to spend a lot of time in the hospital for the first few days. They should be able and instructed to feed, change, and dress their children. They should be encouraged to comfort them, to prepare them for each procedure, to accompany them to X ray, to surgery, to treatment rooms. They need not be included in each treatment, for their presence may unnerve the physician or technician and may prolong the procedure. But then this should be explained to the parent and to the child.

As children begin to recover, become accustomed to the surroundings and realize that their parents have not deserted them, the parents can begin to go home at night. In each case, children should be prepared and warned before the parent leaves. Older children may have little need of their parents in the hospital after the first critical period is over.

What else can make a difference to the emotional outcome of illness and hospitalization? Preparation for each step may be the most critical way of alleviating a child's anxiety. Even though children may still worry and fight about each procedure, they know that there are limits to the pain and the fear involved. By telling children what to expect, adults can give them a way of understanding the steps of the treatment and provide the sense of basic trust, the knowledge that someone cares. Without such preparation, children will be at the mercy of not knowing and of being completely on their own.

Permission to regress, to cry, to fall back on a "lovey" or a thumb can be a real relief. Most children try very hard to be grown up—even in the face of pain and illness. When they fail, they feel it as a personal failure. Parents or hospital personnel who explain the reasons for their "failure" and give a child permission to fail help him to keep fighting at such a time.

In the hospital setting, all experiences that lead to a better understanding of themselves and of

their illnesses become of extra significance.
Learning about their bodies, even about death
itself, can give children a feeling of mastery
which makes illness and pain more tolerable. Play
that involves such situations as nursing
procedures or medical treatment becomes a
therapeutic experience. Many pediatric hospitals
have play specialists who introduce children and
their parents to such play experiences. For
immobilized children, play that gives them a
chance to be aggressive or to master a situation,
becomes an opportunity for feeling in control of
an otherwise debilitating and discouraging
situation.

One of the most therapeutic roles for sick
children is that of caring for someone else. When
they can be out of bed, give them a job of caring
for or reading to or playing with another child. Or
let them help on the ward. When they can
identify with doctors and nurses in protecting and
nurturing other ill children, they are well on the
way to their own recovery.

In the case of a chronically ill child, or even in
an acute illness that frightens the child about its
outcome, providing him or her with another child
of close to the same age with whom to identify
can make a real difference. Children who are
about to undergo cardiac surgery and who are
acutely conscious of the potential for severe
discomfort and even death, latch on greedily to
another child of their age who has been through
and come out of such surgery. I'm sure that this is
true of most other situations as well.

Once children come home, there is an

important opportunity for parents to help them work out their fears and the tensions that have been created by the illness and the hospitalization. Play and talking about the experiences can be of major value. If one sets up a make-believe hospital room, or an operating room with dolls or teddy bears, it can be surprising how much may come to the surface which can be illuminating to the parent about how the child has experienced his or her traumatic experiences. Such an artificially created play situation becomes informative to the parents and therapeutic for the children as they reconstruct their experience and play out their anxiety under the supportive eye of their parents. Here again, one can see the value for the child of having a caring adult present during his or her frightening experience.

The real tragedy of not having pediatric wards set up for parent participation is that parents could learn so much about caring for their sick children while they are still in the hospital. Most parents must flounder at home alone, often using less effective ways of coping and helping the child to cope. Ideally, I would like to see hospital personnel accept parents and children as a unit. There are an increasing number of physicians, of pediatric units, and of nursing schools that understand this, and are making parent participation a priority in the care of sick children. Parents can now choose pediatricians and surgeons who do believe strongly in supporting programs of unlimited visiting and of parent-oriented teaching and pediatric care, and who will go out of their way to request liberal visiting hours or living-in arrangements for parents who can be there. Parents who are well-instructed in the beginning of a child's stay can begin to substitute for understaffed nursing care with their own as well as other children, and indirectly provide much-needed nursing time for critically ill youngsters and for children whose parents cannot live in.

In addition to choosing a physician who is sympathetic and supportive to their involvement in the ill child's care, parents can do a great deal in their role as citizens in demanding better hospital arrangements for parents and children. For we must recognize that children's need for their parents continues and even increases when they are ill and must be hospitalized.

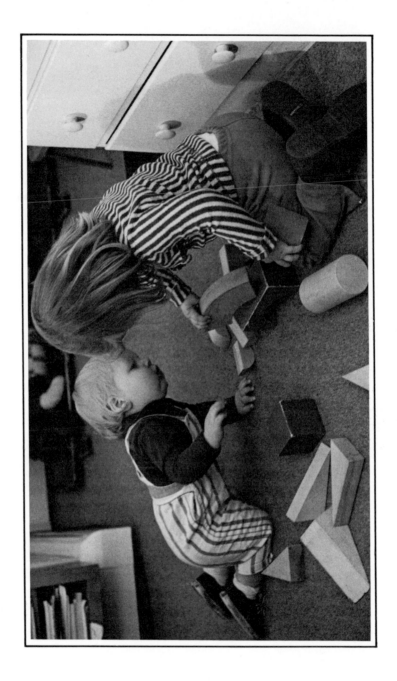

## Chapter 12

# Toys and their meaning for parents and children

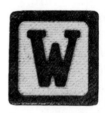hen the earliest crises of infancy are over—colicky crying, feeding difficulties, and so on—parents of three- and four-month-old infants begin to worry about the kinds of toys they should be providing for their babies. One young woman whose husband is a struggling student put into words the thinking of many mothers of babies in this age group: "I realize that I should buy the newest and best toys to provide stimulation for my baby. I want to give him the best chance to learn how to play *early* so he'll be able to keep up with other children his age. We can't afford too many toys, but on the other hand, if it's worth it to push Grant's development, we certainly will find the money somewhere. Many of my friends, already have bought educational toys, and I feel we should too, if as much research as they say has been put into them."

When I asked Mrs. Richards why she and her husband didn't make a cradle toy of squares of colored cardboard to string across Grant's crib so that he could learn to reach for them while he lay in his bed in the mornings, she said, "But my friends buy more complicated toys with many different sizes and shapes. If we just used squares, wouldn't Grant miss out on learning about other shapes?"

As Mrs. Richards talked I became pretty upset. My immediate reaction to her statement was anger at the pressure she felt to respond to the advertising of toy manufacturers. But as I began to think it over, I realized that the manufacturers themselves were responding to a trend that society was creating.

The suggestion that there is a *need* for educational toys is coming from child experts. For a number of years psychologists have been pushing toward earlier cognitive, or intellectual, stimulation, and the implication has been that parents must provide their infants with toys that will "help them learn how to learn." Implicit in this kind of pressure is that children won't learn enough by themselves, that young parents today cannot offer enough stimulation for their tiny babies, that their affectionate play and caring does not provide children with enough necessary building blocks for the future. Implicit too is that parents must be told by experts and toy manufacturers what their baby needs to draw her or him on from one stage of development to the next.

The competitive nature of our society puts

added pressure on young parents. Not only do they feel they must keep up with everyone around them and with all the latest information in the field of child development, but also they feel that, unless they do, their baby may lose a foothold in our society's competitive race.

Of course, I don't agree with this kind of thinking and I don't like the pressure it puts on parents. I am saddened to realize how undermined young mothers and fathers must feel who cannot trust their own instinctive reactions to playing with their baby and who feel they must be told how to teach a four-month-old to compete in our world. After talking with Mrs. Richards, I had to realize that young parents today are getting a real brainwashing about the importance of early cognitive development.

Research has been widely quoted that seems to establish the importance of providing children with early cognitive stimulation. But this research has been done with groups of really deprived children. For the most part these children were in institutions that were unable to provide the person-to-person contact they needed. And even when parents were available, they often were too deprived and disorganized themselves to be able to see the needs of their babies, too desolate to provide even simple homemade toys.

When the researchers came into such environments to carry out their studies, the effect of their efforts was to organize the disor-ganization, to fill the emptiness. As a result of the caring attitudes brought by the researchers, as much as because of the toys they offered, the environment could provide a new kind of responsiveness that filled the children's desperate need. It's no wonder that they thrived!

But the conditions of deprivation that were improved by toys and stimulation were not present in Grant's case. His family cared about him, played with him, and provided him with all he needed, both emotionally and cognitively. Certainly he didn't need complex toys to supplement any deficiency. And I felt that Mrs. Richards would be wasting her money and devaluing her own good parenting by thinking she ought to provide them.

What little extra stimulation Grant might have used certainly could be provided by a set of multicolored cardboard squares! And the main thing the simple homemade toy would represent was a chance to play alone when his parents, who cared a lot and were available to him most of his day, needed time to themselves. He could learn to master his own new skills and to feel the excitement of self-mastery—a feeling that is the base of all learning. What kind of toy he learns this from may be of relatively little importance in an environment that offers as much as Grant's does in care and affection.

Through play, children learn about themselves as well as about the world around them. They may learn about their intellectual competence in one kind of play, about their emotional competence in another, and about motor skills in another—or they may combine all three kinds of learning in one afternoon of play. But the seriousness of the goal—learning about oneself

and how to grow up in an adult world—certainly
cannot be ignored.

As two children play beside each other, they
learn how a peer sees other men and women of
the culture. They imitate one parent and discard
parts of his or her behavior, and then imitate the
other and decide *in play* what aspects of each
parent they want as a permanent part of their
own personality. Their peers are a good testing
ground for the new behaviors before they are
fully accepted. As the play becomes more involved
and the children begin to act out more aggressive
behavior, it is easy to see that this kind of role
playing and testing of self is serious business.

One of my colleagues, Daniel G. Freedman, at
the University of Chicago, demonstrated the
serious aspect of play with little boys. After being
introduced to my four-year-old and his friend of
the same age, he asked, "Which of you is
stronger?" Both children replied simultaneously,
"I am," and locked in each other's arms to prove
it. When neither prevailed, they began to climb
high on the jungle gym and then to run up and
down the street, each in an effort to outdo the
other. Finally exhausted, they came back to us,
having worn themselves out trying to answer the
question.

If one accepts learning about oneself and about
the world as a goal for play, what role do toys
serve? Wouldn't children learn more about
themselves if they had to make their own toys?
Certainly the ingenuity of a child's imagination is
demonstrated even when adults don't provide toys.
Babies left in a cradle under a tree will reach up

for leaves to bat at with clumsy fists. They will watch a bee buzz around the cradle when no mobile has been offered.

In one of the less affluent societies I have visited, where no ready-made toys were available, I remember watching a group of three-year-old children play with the substitutes they themselves had constructed. A forked stick holding a smaller stick became a mother and baby and a tall stick represented the father.

Certainly it seems to me that when children make their own toys, or when parents help their children do so, it always produces the most gratifying results. Still, Elaine Gurion, who teaches mothers how to make ingenious toys from recycled materials at the Boston Children's Museum, has told me that she finds painfully few mothers who dare compare their homemade efforts to manufactured toys. If this is true, we certainly are not fostering one of the most valuable aspects of toys for small children—that they can represent a form of communication. Toys that are made by parents immediately become invested with all the magic that parents have to offer their children.

This is not to say that commercial toys have no value—they certainly do! First of all, many of them can offer a child a kind of excitement and complexity that homemade toys sometimes cannot. And then, of course, most of them have been designed according to rigid standards of safety.

At the same time, in a society as complex as ours commercial toys can become important

adjuncts for learning. And most important, they
may serve a major role in providing and
reinforcing communication with others—peers,
siblings, and parents. This role is a valuable one,
and one with which we can afford to be honestly
concerned.

For example, many toys have labels and
instruction booklets that tell parents how to play
with the child with the toy. This may sound pretty
condescending, yet as a distractible father I have
experienced the value of an instruction booklet
that came with a racing toy. The booklet
described ways to race the toy, from which I could
find enough complexity to satisfy me, and there
was enough simplicity in its wording to give my
children an understanding of how to "gang up on
and beat Daddy." We relied on its instructions as
ways of testing each other, of conquering our
internal struggles as a family, of stirring up new
roles for and new competition with each other, of
having fun with each other at many levels.

I do not feel that labels or instructions are a
substitute for interpersonal exploration. But I can
see that a busy parent may want them to help
him or her decide which toy will reward him or
her and the small child simultaneously, so that
the result of a period of play together will be one
of communicating with and learning about the
other.

I would hope that toys would increase the
chances for periods of play—however short—
between a busy parent and a parent-hungry child.
Too many of us feel guilty that we haven't time
for our children—when it may not be quantity,

but quality, of time with them that we have as a goal. Can toys make such bridges for us? If they can, they are worth the effort for all of us.

One young father expressed his own involvement in an "educational toy" that was accompanied by a brochure explaining the stage of development of his year-old-baby. He said, "Janet may not be learning much by stacking those colored blocks on top of one another in the right sequence, but I am. When I see her pick up one, compare it to another, and discard it for the next one in sequence, I get a real charge! I feel like I've created a genius and that she's learning by herself all the things I'd like to be able to teach her. And I've done it! I could sit and watch her by the hour."

I asked him how much the brochure had added to this pleasure. He replied that probably he never would have known how to look at his baby's play or what to see without these guidelines on her stage of development.

I'm not sure I agree with this father's estimate of the brochure's importance, and I have seen parents overuse the knowledge they have gained from such things in an effort to push the child's development along, but I am sure that the cementing of the parent-child relationship is the most important ingredient in this episode. How much cement the toy manufacturer has provided may be open to question, but the fact that such a potential exists is indisputable.

But there are other issues that are not really so clear. For example, can toys be so rigidly structured with advice and labels that they are no longer any fun? If labels tell children what to expect, and parents buy them for their "fit" with the child's stage of development and temperament, couldn't we inadvertently be cutting out the factor of surprise and exploration and creating a dullness that might lead to boredom? Couldn't we thereby be encouraging parents to believe that such products offered enough stimulation, and thus to abdicate their roles in play with their babies? Couldn't toys in our culture become substitutes for play with people?

How do we see to it that the toy manufacturers and child experts do not intimidate mothers and fathers so that they buy expensive and unnecessary products, and how do we at the same time reinforce parents' natural authority in filling their children's needs?

The manufacturers are spending vast sums on good research, but paradoxically this laudable effort, whose end is, of course, business success, is not all that is required. It seems to me that some kind of multidisciplinary advisory group ought to be formed so that there can be more formal communication between the manufacturers and the psychologists, pediatricians, government representatives, and consumer advocates. The knowledge about toys and their influence on children's development that could be assimilated in this way might be extremely important.

I think the most important goal of the toy manufacturers, of the parental groups, and of the professionals who might become interested in this venture would be to encourage parents to use toys to have more fun with their children. I am all for that!

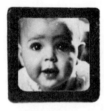

# What to look for in toys

1.  Is the toy worth the price? Will it hold your child's attention beyond Christmas Day? An expensive toy should be made to last and provide enjoyment over a long period.
2.  Does your child expect too much from the toy? Often children are bitterly disappointed when they actually see the television toy they wanted so desperately. Sit down with them on Saturday morning and see how the toys are advertised. Compare this with products in the stores.
3.  Is your child the right age for the toy? Television ads rarely mention an age range— after all, Saturday-morning programs are geared to a "two-to-eleven-year-old" audience, network executives tell us.
4.  Does the toy have batteries or complicated mechanical parts? Remember—these are the first things to go wrong.
5.  Is the toy safe? Sadly, only you can judge whether or not a toy is safe. There is a Child Protection and Toy Safety Act on the books, but it is poorly enforced. Be wary of toys that require electricity (one toy stove reached temperatures of over 300 degrees), shoot objects

in the air, or have sharp edges or unfinished surfaces that could hurt your child. Small children try to put things in their mouths, so be wary of loose parts. Think of how a child might misuse the toy.

The newly created Consumer Product Safety Commission of the federal government has begun to check on unsafe banned toys in the stores, using consumers to do the investigating, and promises to serve as an active watchdog in the area of product safety. The Food and Drug Administration also lists dangerous toys on occasion and a List of Banned Products is available from their Consumer Information Center.

# Index

ACTION, 206
Action for Children's Television, 190–95
Adenoidal surgery, 197–98
Adolescents and pediatrician, 21
Advertising
 and educational toys, 222
 effect on children, 192–95
American Academy of Pediatrics, 78
Amphetamines, 99
Anesthesia, *See* Drugs and medication
Anxiety
 child-doctor relationship, 15–20
 and childbirth drugs, 23, 26, 31–33
 and disciplining, 113, 116–20
 and hospitalization, 200, 210–11, 215
 with new babies, xx–xxi, 56–57
 parental, 4–6, 31–32, 37
 and sibling jealousy, 166–67
Apgar score, 28–29
Association for Child Care in Hospitals, 209

Babies, *See* Infants; Newborn babies
"Baby-proofing," 113–17
Bed-wetting, 133, 139–40, 144–47, 208, 211
Boston Children's Medical Center, 200
Boston Children's Museum, 199, 226
Bowel movements, 131–32, 135–36, 147–49
Bowlby, John, 32, 210, 212
Brain damage, 98–99
Breast-feeding, 52–53, 56, 62, 65
 and drugs, 33–34, 36

Childbirth
 and drugs, 23–39
 natural, 24–27

Childbirth Education Association, xxii
Child Protection and Toy Safety Act, 230
Child psychiatry, xviii–xx, 86–87, 99
Children
 fathers and, 8–11
 institutionalized, 76–77, 223–24
 and pediatrician, 5–7, 13–21
 use of sibling rivalry, 175–77
Children in Hospitals, 204, 209–10
Colic, 50, 59–71
 cause of, 65
 solutions, 65–71
Constipation, 131, 138, 140, 142
 cause and treatment, 147–49
Consumer Product Safety Commission, 231
"Contingent reinforcement," 86–87
Crying, 49–51, 56, 92
 normal period of, 67, 69–70
 and pain, 205

Depression, *See* Post-partum depression
Discipline, 111–27; goals of, 123–24
 and permissiveness, 116–17
"Disintegration of the ego," 181–82
Drugs and medication
 for childbirth, 23–39
 effect on mother, 31
 effect on newborn, 29–31
 for hyperactive children, 99

"Electric Company, The" (television program), 185
Environment of infant, 73–89
 and toys, 223–24
Erikson, Eric, 153

*Family Guide to Children's Television, The* (Kaye), 193–95
Fathers
 and childbirth, 35, 37–41